# PASS YOUR ORAL OB/GYN BOARD EXAM!

• How to Prepare for it • How to Take it • How to Pass It!

## Anita Krishna Das, MD FACOG

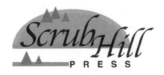

**Publisher's Cataloging-in-Publication Data**

Das, Anita Krishna.

Pass your oral ob/gyn board exam! / Anita Krishna Das, MD, FACOG.

p.   cm.

ISBN: 978-0-98229-212-9

1. Obstetrics—Examinations, questions, etc. 2. Gynecology—Examinations, questions, etc.

R834.5 .D37 2009

618—dc22                                                                 2009922945

Publisher: Scrub Hill Press, Inc.

Cover Design: Robert Johnson, Johnson Design

Interior Design: Shawn Morningstar

Editorial Assistance: Mim Eisenberg, WordCraft

10  9  8  7  6  5  4  3  2

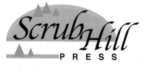

46 South Glebe Road
Suite 301
Arlington, VA 22204
800 516 1088
www.scrubhill.com

*I am forever grateful to my family, Alex, Austin, and Paul. Without their support, this book, let alone the fourth edition, would not be possible nor worthwhile.*

# Table of Contents

# Preface

The failure of one of our glowing junior faculty members to pass his oral OB/GYN board exam scared me into thinking about the exam the last year of my residency. I knew I was going to practice in a town remote from an academic center, so I figured I had better get all the help I could while still under the protective cloak of a knowledgeable faculty.

My bubble was burst. I asked everyone, and they hardly knew anything about the exam. I couldn't find much on the subject matter (other than "Know everything"), the process ("I've repressed all of that"), or the conduct of the exam ("They grill you under the hot white lights"). Logically, I turned to graduates who had recently taken the exam. The little information I unearthed was inconsistent.

I was worried, but life got busy with finishing residency, moving, and joining a practice. I was hopeful that my uneasiness would wane after I began the process and that my worries would be for naught. I was wrong. The ABOG guidelines were vague and generic. I was lost and overwhelmed about how or where to begin.

I dedicated a year and a half to preparing for the exam. Life got put on hold. I have never prepared so hard for a test. But I was ready.

During the exam, I knew my stuff. Yet the examiners were skilled at leaving a fragment of doubt with most questions. By the end of the exam, I didn't know if I had passed. I was outraged. I knew I really knew my stuff, and no one deserved to pass more than me. Fortunately, I received my congratulatory letter in just three days, so I was not in agony for long. As I read the letter, I was flooded with relief, but then my anger began to swell. I threw down the letter and cried, "There has to be a better way."

I had learned so much about the process of preparing for and taking the exam that I felt compelled to share it. Fortuitously, the medical school in the state where I practiced did not have an OB/GYN residency, so I linked up with a national review course. As I shared my experiences throughout the country, two things happened. The first was that I was able to tap into the target audience and accumulate a huge pool of feedback about exam experiences. Second, because there are so few resources on the topic, I was inundated with appreciation and encouraged to make this information more widely available.

This fourth edition updates recent numerous changes in exam topics and format. There is a continued trend toward standardizing the test. Currently. the exam consists of only the case list and the case of the days. The case of the day chapter is greatly expanded with past exam recollections. Interesting that the fourth edition reflects already the pendulum swinging back toward the philosophy in the first edition, in that finally we're back to being specialists rather than primary care doctors.

The fourth edition also marks my nearly two decades of mentoring physicians seeking their board certification. I marvel that the approach recommended in the first edition has stood the test of time. Of course, I have fine tuned it throughout the years, but this approach is really quite simple, and perhaps that's the reason for its success.

This book will help you to organize and prioritize your studies, but you will still have to roll up your sleeves and learn the stuff cold. Please consider my advice on how to construct your case list most carefully. A well constructed case list makes all the difference in its defense. This book will also reduce your anxiety about taking the exam, but you still have to practice, practice, practice with mock orals to get proficient with the oral exam format.

I am readily available to assist you throughout the entire process. You may reach me through krisdas@earthlink.net or krisdas@mchsi.com. You may call 1-877-ABC-OBGYN or go through www.americasboardreview.com for my phone numbers.

I hope this book is a compass for you. May it give you the shortest and easiest path to board certification. Good luck!

A. Krishna Das, MD, FACOG
April 2009

# Chapter

# The Oral Versus the Written Exam: How They Differ

The most common test format throughout medical school and residency is a written exam. Years of experience with the written format make taking the written exam for Phase I of the boards straightforward and predictable. Preparing for and taking an oral exam, however, are quite different. Experimentation with the oral exam format should not be reserved for your first encounter with the oral boards, the most important test of your career.

The oral boards differ from the written exam in several ways. The first is **timing**. You cannot sit for the oral exam until you have successfully completed the written exam. Most graduates have transitioned into clinical practice. This is just enough time to fall out of the mandatory rigors of the academic environment of residency. No more morning report, morbidity and mortality conference, or grand rounds—just enough time to have succumbed to "the good life," just enough time to "get out of shape" for intense academic discipline. This academic apathy results in a rude awakening when you face the intensity of effort that will be required to prepare adequately for the oral exam.

Isolation from the medical center mecca not only predisposes to academic laxity but also strips away the advantage of "misery loves company" that helps to motivate studying. Typically residents prepare collectively for upcoming tests, such as CREOG (Council on Resident Education in Obstetrics and Gynecology) in-service exams and the written board exam.

At a minimum there is sharing of knowledge about the test. Often there are even formal study groups. Furthermore, staff mentors are eager to share knowledge gained from previous residents' experience. After all, the program's reputation is at stake. Poor performance on standardized tests is a reflection of the staff's mentoring. The group's efforts culminate in the written exam at the end of residency.

Upon graduation from residency and successful completion of the written boards, active candidates migrate to all corners of the country. Most have joined practices with senior partners who have already completed the oral exam process. Thus the severing of academic ties strips away the familiar comfort of camaraderie as you tackle the oral exam.

For the first time, and unfortunately for the biggest test of our career, most of us have no idea of the format, let alone the test topics. The familiarity of a written exam is gone, and you are all alone. Most commonly, the residency programs do nothing to prepare you for what's to come. Thus, most of us lacked foresight and insight during residency to tap into the faculty's knowledge about the oral exam. Most residents cannot or refuse to see past the written exam; after all, you can't even sit for the orals until you pass the written board exam.

So now you're isolated. Your partners and local colleagues can't remember (or purposely repressed) the details you need. Your out-of-town resident colleagues don't know any more than you. The feeling of impending doom and panic sets in.

Yet the biggest obstacle of all is **time**. Everybody competes for your time. Residency is no longer an acceptable excuse. Family, social, civic, and church demands—let alone your practice—make finding time to prepare for the exam almost humanly impossible.

Besides timing, another major difference between the oral and the written boards is **format**. The purpose of the written exam is to confirm a foundation in the basic sciences. On the other hand, the oral exam establishes the ability to apply that basic knowledge to patient care.

Successful performance on the written exam is no guarantee of similar success with the oral exam. Unlike for a written exam, regurgitation of isolated facts is not good enough. Furthermore, selection of the "right" answer is only the beginning, not the end, in the oral exam. You must be able to substantiate your answers unhesitatingly.

Finally, the oral exam has an **impact** on your career. The significance of "needing" to pass the oral exam has changed. Customarily, everyone has to take, but not pass, the written boards to graduate from residency. Thank heaven! However, you don't have to be board-certified to practice medicine. Historically, board certification is a feather in your cap, a mark of prestigious academic excellence.

Thanks to managed care, Joint Commission, and CMS (Centers for Medicare & Medicaid Services) all of that has changed. Board certification is now required for many managed care panels, hospital staff privileges, and group practice employment. You can still practice medicine without board certification—but not how or where you want to. Thus, more is at stake with the oral exam—maybe everything.

In conclusion, the oral exam differs from the written exam in its timing, format, and impact on your ability to practice medicine. The task of preparing for the oral board exam is enormous. There are no shortcuts. As an anonymous philosopher observed, "The only place where success comes before work is in the dictionary." In contrast to the written exam, a photographic memory affords little advantage. Finally, hard work is rewarded. With the oral exam you truly get out of it what you put into it. Testimonials from those who have failed repeatedly confirm this observation.

The task is surmountable. The entire elephant can be eaten, but only one bite at a time. The following chapters will tell you how. Get out your fork and knife, and come with a ravenous appetite. Bon appétit!

# 2

## Chapter

# The Application Process

## Applying for the Exam: Fast Track vs. Traditional

The *Bulletin* published by the American Board of Obstetrics and Gynecology, Inc. is a guideline for the application process. You will refer to this invaluable resource repeatedly throughout the entire process. You may request a copy from the Board office or download one from their website at **www.abog.org**.

Since 2002, candidates can apply for the accelerated oral exam process. Historically, you had to wait two years between successful completions of the written exam and the oral exam. In 2002 this was shortened to one year.

There are pros and cons for each track. The advantage of the fast track is you get it over with sooner. Why put off until tomorrow what you can do today? You also can ride on the academic momentum of your written exam preparation, rather than letting it slide away for another year.

The advantage of the traditional track is that it's logistically easier. You get a whole year to get settled into your new practice, community, lifestyle, etc. With the fast track, you have to begin collecting cases within a week after completing the written exam. Furthermore, the exponential growth in your clinical skills during the first couple of years in practice will really help you on the exam. For this reason, I recommend the traditional track.

I recommend the fast track **only** if you are immediately starting into a practice limited to just obstetrics or gynecology or you are planning to pursue subspecialty fellowship training. Since you are examined in **both** topics, you won't forget as much in one year. However, you will need to use cases from your chief year in the off subject. In other words, if you are joining a GYN-only practice, you will need to use obstetrical patients from your chief residency year for your obstetrics case list. Obviously, this will be a piece of cake if you are reading this in your residency and you now know to **save that log**! If you are having an "oops" moment and realized you gleefully pitched it when you were cleaning out the chief resident's desk, then begin to make arrangements **now** to recapture that data.

If you choose the "fast track," you must return your oral exam application (sent with your written exam results) along with your application fee or go online to **www.abog.org** by September 15 of the year preceding the oral exam. You will be notified by October 1 if you are accepted into the accelerated process. Thereafter, you must then meet the same requirements as the other candidates.

If you do not want to do the fast track, then the application form for the oral exam may be requested online at **www.abog.org**. Traditionally, you could not obtain the application until November 1 of the year preceding the exam. Thus, if your exam is in 2010, the form may be requested no earlier than November 1, 2009. Effective 2009, ABOG pushed it even further, to February 1. Whether it's November or, worse yet, February, your case list collection should have began many months earlier in July. Thus, I recommend that you request a packet or case list software from the preceding year so that you can begin your case list data entry promptly in July. A delay of four or, worse yet, eight months until November or February makes it overwhelmingly difficult to catch up with the backlog of data entry. The only risk of using the preceding year's forms is the unlikely chance that the format will change four months later when you order your "official" packet.

The completed application form, the application fee, a copy of each current medical license, and two passport-sized (2 inches x 2 inches) photographs (with the candidate's signature across the front) must be received on or before March 15 of the year of the exam. A late fee is charged for applications received from March 16 to April 15, and there is an even steeper fee for applications received between April 16 to April 30. No applications are accepted after April 30. If your application (not necessarily your case list) is accepted, then you will be notified in July. Once you are notified in July of your admissibility to the oral exam, you must send an examination fee and your case list by August 1. You can submit your case list as late as August 14, but you will of course be assessed a late fine. No case lists or examination fees are accepted after August 14.

## Requirements

The ABOG *Bulletin* lists the requirements to sit for the exam. Only the highlights are discussed below:

1. A passing grade on the written exam no longer than five years before the oral exam.

2. You cannot be involved in litigation or investigation regarding practice activities, or ethical or moral issues.

3. Unrestricted license to practice medicine in the United States or its territories or a province of Canada since at least June 1 of the year preceding the exam. Candidates practicing in any other country must submit a letter from a senior officer from their hospital(s), verifying their credentials.

4. Active engagement in an unsupervised practice, which is defined as: independent, continuous, unsupervised patient care *limited* to obstetrics and gynecology from July 1 of the year preceding the exam through June 30 of the year of the exam. Time spent in a fellowship does not meet this requirement.

5. Practice that consists exclusively of ambulatory care is not considered adequate.

6. If your medical license or hospital practice has ever been restricted or revoked, a written explanation of the circumstances must accompany the application.

7. Submission of a case list.

## Notification of Acceptance

You will be notified in July or October of the year of your exam if your application is accepted for the traditional or fast track, respectively. You must submit your case list by August 1. If it is approved by the Board, you will be notified at least one month in advance of the date and time of your exam.

## Limitations

You must pass the oral exam within six years of passing the written exam (unless serving in a board-approved fellowship). You may take the oral exam only three times. If you fail the oral exam three times or do not pass the oral exam within six years, you must repeat and pass the written exam before you can take the oral exam again. There is no limit to the number of times the written exam and the six-year cycle to pass the oral exam can be repeated.

## Qualifications

Candidates must be of good moral and ethical character. Your character may be verified by inquiry to administrative officers of organizations and institutions to whom your mode of practice is known. Further-more, time spent in a teaching or research position that does not provide sufficient evidence of independent, continuous, and unsupervised responsibility for patient care is not permissible. Falsification of data (including case lists) or evidence of other "professional misbehavior" may result in deferral of a candidate's application for at least three years.

## Chapter

# Scope of the Exam

The purpose of the exam is to evaluate your knowledge and skills in solving clinical problems in obstetrics, gynecology, and women's health. Most importantly, you are expected to demonstrate a level of competence that allows you to serve as a consultant to non-OB/GYNs in your community.

There is no better DNA of a practitioner's mode of practice than his case list. This is the one component of the exam that has remained constant for many years. Thus, half of your test is spent defending your case list. You must demonstrate the following abilities when questioned from your case list:

1. To develop a diagnosis, including the necessary clinical, laboratory, and diagnostic procedures

2. To select and apply proper treatment under elective and emergency conditions

3. To prevent, recognize, and manage complications

4. To plan and direct follow-up and continuing care

The *Bulletin* clearly states that the case list is an essential component of the test. However, they are quite vague as to the other components. The *Bulletin* simply states that "other clinical problems will be included with possible visual aids." In the past, this has included interpretation of sonograms, operative videos, and video graphics of various conditions. However, since 2007 the other half has been exclusively the structured cases or "case of the day."

This vague yet all-encompassing subject matter makes studying rather challenging. In contrast to the written exam, for which extensive lists of test topics are available, the only list for the oral exam is each of the case list categories. The tight-lipped examiners have done well to squelch leakage of similar knowledge about the oral exam. The contents of the exam and the criteria by which you pass or fail are their best-kept secrets. Such knowledge exists primarily from exam recall of previous candidates. The feedback to candidates who fail is characteristically noncommittal. The ABOG Diplomate states only that "the mode of practice continues to be the major reason for failure."

Your chances of passing the exam are excellent. ABOG reports that the pass rates for all candidates from 1990 to 2007 have a narrow range of 83–87%. American graduates fare best; typically, 85% pass the first time. Approximately 65–75% of international graduates pass the first time. These statistics, however, are skewed and falsely reassuring. Usually, only the best-prepared candidates sit for the exam. Because most candidates have invested at least 16 months of preparation, they represent "survival of the fittest." Thus, only the best need apply—that is, until recently.

The advent of managed care and CMS's pay for performance will lead to a new set of statistics. Symbolically, board certification has been a prestigious badge of academic excellence. Such accolades, however, were not necessary to practice medicine—until now. Increasingly only board-certified physicians are selected as providers for HMOs and similar insurance groups. Consequently, both hospitals and group practices are forced to require the same of their staff. Board certification has become mandatory to ensure financial livelihood.

As less prepared candidates begin to apply for the exam, the statistics will surely change. Most likely the pass rate will decline. Certainly, we will then have a deeper appreciation of just how challenging the oral exam truly is.

# 4

## Chapter

# Getting Started

## Priority of Study Topics

The oral exam can cover any topic related to obstetrics, gynecology, and women's health. Obviously, however, it is impossible to review every topic. Perhaps the most common and costly mistake is failure to prioritize and focus your studying.

To prioritize, you must identify your personal strengths and weaknesses in specific topics. It is neither helpful nor realistic—yet typical of most compulsive physicians—to underestimate your strengths. Most candidates assume that they are weak or at least need to review all topics. The task of identifying and then prioritizing your knowledge base entails two critical steps.

**The first step**—and the most influential on prioritizing—is to identify which topics are most likely to appear on the exam. Fortunately, the test lasts for only a finite period; thus, only a finite number of topics can be covered. It is surprisingly easy to predict the likelihood that a topic will appear on the exam. Based on candidates' recollection of past exam topics, certain topics predictably appear year after year. Such a priceless list is covered in Chapter 8: Studying for the Exam.

Topics raised by your case list are also likely contenders. How to extrapolate which of these topics is most likely to appear is covered in Chapter 5: The Case List.

**The second step** is to identify your individual strengths and weaknesses in topics not yet covered. Although there are as many different ways to tackle this problem as there are candidates, two techniques are popular.

The common features of these two techniques are to be candid with your critique, to limit time and resources, and to revise your list periodically.

The first method is to take your OB/GYN textbooks and skim their table of contents for broad subject areas. For areas that you identify as your weaknesses, skim further through the chapter for specific topics. The second method is to attend a review course approximately six months before the exam. Prior to the course, you should make three lists categorizing topics as top, medium, and low priority. As the lectures proceed, fill in the various topics on the respective lists.

The time spent in identifying your study priorities before you actually begin studying is well worth the time invested. You will markedly enhance your efficiency in the remaining study time. More importantly, however, you will cover first the topics that are most likely to occur on your exam.

## References

Certainly, there are as many different references and resources as there are candidates. The most important variable in selecting your resources is to recognize that your goal is to *review* the topic. Failure to discipline yourself and to limit your review is the most common reason for running out of time to cover all of the topics on your priority study list.

The best safeguard is to select resources that are limited to a review of topics. Thus, the last reference to choose is a textbook, because its purpose is to provide an in-depth and exhaustive treatise of specific topics. Even so, the number of qualifying references is vast. Feedback from previous successful candidates, however, consistently reveals a consensus on three sources. All are ACOG publications that represent the standard of care by which you are judged.

The first is *Precis*, an ACOG publication that is a concise summary of individual topics in OB/GYN. This reference is short and sweet and provides an excellent review in a time-efficient manner. The text is written from a patient management perspective, which is exactly the style for the oral board exam.

The second reference is the *PROLOG* series. PROLOG is an acronym for Personal Review of Learning on Obstetrics and Gynecology. These reviews consist of clinically oriented, multiple-choice questions with an editorial discussion of the answer. Although geared toward a written exam format, the books in the *PROLOG* series are an excellent source to judge your proficiency in individual topics. They can be used in the beginning to assist in identifying study topics or at the end of a review to verify its thoroughness.

The final recommended resource is the ACOG *Compendium*. As its name implies, it is a compilation of clinical practice guidelines. It consists of *Committee Opinions, Practice (Educational) Bulletins, Policy Statements,* and *Technology Assessments.*

The ACOG *Committee Opinions* are briefs about "clinical issues of an urgent or emergent nature" or "non-clinical topics such as policy, economics, and social issues." They represent ACOG's stance on the hottest controversial issues confronting practitioners. Reference to these briefs during the exam substantiates a candidate's course of action, particularly if it deviates from the examiner's opinion.

*Policy Statements* are just that. They are the College's position on key issues approved by the executive board. If you choose to practice contrary to the ACOG's position, then you definitely want to be able to defend why you are swimming against the current.

*Technology Assessments* describe specific technologies and their application. You should be familiar with these as the national standard of care, especially if you provide such services. The most common is ultrasound, a useful tool we use daily, whether performed by ourselves or our technician. It is so commonplace that we often take for granted the science behind the technology and quality control measures. Both are hot test topics.

*Practice Bulletins* (successor to the *Educational Bulletins*) are evidence-based practice guidelines. They are the final answer on any issue since they are based on sound, peer-reviewed clinical research. They represent ACOG's recommendations and henceforth should be also your preferred method of diagnosis and management of a condition. They are *the* best source for a brief, to-the-point, clinical review of specific topics. Unquestionably, you should start your review of every topic with the corresponding *Practice (Educational) Bulletin*; hopefully, you will also be able to end it there also.

The bottom line in selecting your references is to limit them. Choose resources that are restricted to a *review* of the topic. Textbooks are a last resort and should be used sparingly.

## Review Courses

Let's first make sure we're on the same sheet of music by defining a review course. A review course consists of multiple days (usually at least five) of didactic lectures covering a review of a wide spectrum of OB/GYN topics by multiple faculty, both generalists and subspecialists. This is not to be confused with a tutorial service or seminars that deceptively use the name review course.

Review courses are helpful for several reasons. They allow a pace and intensity of review that are difficult to match with independent study. Furthermore, they are an excellent means to prioritize study topics. Perhaps most important, however, is the "step-away" time that allows you to focus exclusively on studying. Several variables should be considered in selecting a course.

The reputation of a review course is a good place to start. Ask your colleagues what course(s) they attended. What was their reason for choosing that course? How long ago did they attend? Most important, would they attend it again and would they highly recommend it for you? This is a starting point, but you need to do your due diligence to verify their recommendations match your needs.

The first consideration in choosing a review course is when to attend. Ideally, you should attend one just as you complete your case list collection in May or June of the year of the exam. This timing has two distinct advantages: (1) it is the ideal time to prioritize your study topics and draft a study plan, and (2) it allows optimal incorporation of the strategy that you learned in organizing the case list. As discussed before, half the exam is based on the case list, and the majority of failures are due to inadequate defense. Because the time from the end of the case list compilation (June 30) to the deadline for turning it in (August 1) is so tight, you must have a definite plan to act quickly and efficiently to pursue your strategy.

Another strategic time to enroll in a review course is just before you start your intense studying, which is about two or three months before the exam. You should choose a course that covers the topics that you have already identified as priorities. The course should also address overlooked topics and topics that should be upgraded in priority.

The final opportune time to attend a review course is one or two weeks before the exam. The primary objective is to get into the mind-set for the test: to eat, drink, and sleep OB/GYN. The goal is simply to refresh previously studied topics. If you take the course at any earlier time (even a month before the exam), it is difficult to maintain the intensity and recall necessary for the test. This timing also affords the opportunity to "put it all together" by taking mock oral exams. Recall the steep slope of the learning curve. In learning a new task, you improve dramatically with each repetition. Since few candidates are experienced with the oral exam format, you will markedly improve your performance and your chance of passing by taking even only three mock orals. To walk into the oral exam cold, without having practiced specifically the oral exam format, is a foolish risk and potential waste of months of preparation.

In addition to timing, other factors in selecting a review course should be considered. First and foremost, verify that the course is geared toward the oral exam. The name of the review course should state "**Board** review course," to distinguish it from general review courses. The timing of the course relative to the exam determines which features are offered. Certainly, some lectures should be dedicated to exam strategy. Both didactic and private sessions on the case list should be offered. Verify that the course provides strategy for case list collection, organization, and defense. Take advantage of private tutoring dedicated to your case list alone. Unquestionably, any course offered at least two to three months before the test must offer mock oral exams. If it does not, look for one that does.

Expense is also a consideration. Those review courses that offer a refund of the registration fee if you do not pass your exam cater specifically to those preparing for an exam, and not just those looking for a general review. However, make sure you look at the fine print, as there are usually contingencies in order to receive your refund. The tuition or registration may be only just the beginning. Look for hidden expenses that can put you over budget.

I recommend you consider the following expenses:

**Registration fee:**
> Do they offer a discount for
>> resident/fellow physicians in training?
>>
>> multiple registrants?
>>
>> early registration?
>>
>> armed forces members?
>>
>> returning registrant?
>
> Does it include meals and snacks?

**Lodging:**

Does room rate include:

complementary shuttle to/from airport?

complimentary meals?

What amenities are available:

in-room meal prep (kitchenette, microwave, fridge, etc.)?

on-site or nearby restaurants?

suite to keep studying separate from sleeping?

fitness center?

business center?

swimming pool?

Complimentary shuttle to nearby restaurants, shopping, etc.

Is it safe? Can you go out for a walk or run?

Internet access?

**To save money, consider:**

Sharing with a colleague to cut costs.

Is it less expensive to stay at a different hotel and travel back and forth for lectures?

Bottom line, this is not a vacation conference. All day and often the early evenings are spent in lectures or coaching sessions. Have your family accompany you only if they are keenly aware of your time commitments.

The length of the course is important. Realistically, how long can you stay focused? Most of us have not had to sit **all** day and be lectured to since medical school. Although you will find this surprisingly enjoyable at first, your back and bladder are unconditioned, and both your physical and intellectual stamina quickly falter within a few days. Emotionally, it's also a rude awakening to acknowledge just how much you have forgotten and what a monumental task it will take to get back up to speed. Furthermore, how much time can you afford to be away from your practice or residency? You must budget not just for the time needed for one, but perhaps several courses, as well as for family (remember them?). Thus, I recommend you attend a five-to-seven-day course. Ideally, a course that overlaps with a weekend will minimize time away from your practice. Better yet, perhaps you can couple the review course with a one-to-three-day tutorial course.

Finally, the faculty and the course agenda are the most variable features among different courses. Because the goal is to review, it is not necessary—and actually maybe a waste of time—to have noted academicians as faculty members. They have a tendency to include trivia and to focus on their latest research. The lecturers should focus on patient management issues consistent with the ACOG standards.

The course's promotional material (written and online) mailer or website should boast about the caliber of the faculty, not just their expertise in the topic but also their ability and experience as speakers. Be wary of courses that primarily use residents, fellows, and junior faculty all from the same institution. Chances are they were assigned the topic, so the data they present will promote that institution's, and not necessarily ACOG's, perspective. You should have time with the faculty for questions and especially mock oral exams and case list review. All the speakers must be clinicians. The oral exam is the ultimate clinical application of knowledge. If the review course faculty aren't in the OR, office, or labor and delivery daily, then they have **no** business lecturing on the topic nor giving you advice.

Furthermore, because it is impossible to cover every topic, each course will have a different agenda. Direct inquiry to the course administration should confirm their strategy. The right answer is that the topics were chosen based entirely on the likelihood of occurring on your exam. Refer to Chapter 8: Studying for the Exam, for a list of the "Know Cold" and "Hot Topics" as a list to cross reference with their topics.

Perhaps the most helpful tool for evaluating review courses is through the Internet. With a few key strokes you can conduct a quick, easy, yet thorough comparison of what is currently available. I would start with key search terms, including "OB/GYN board review course" or "OB/GYN review course." A course's website, just like your case list, is an excellent thumbprint as to its philosophy. What is its attention to detail? Is the website current? Is it easy to navigate? Do the testimonials seem sincere and legitimate? Do you feel like you're being swindled? Is there a link designated for faculty or are they relegated to the miscellaneous tab? Can you register online? How quickly does the staff respond to your e-mail inquiries?

Many review courses are available on DVD and/or CD. You should not use these in lieu of attending a course. The substitute is never as good as the real thing. Attendance demands your complete attention and allows for interaction with both faculty and colleagues. Unless the course was just recorded, the DVDs and CDs do not reflect the most recent updates, nor do they often contain evening sessions on exam tips and strategy. However, they are an excellent resource to solidify and reinforce your studies. An excellent-quality DVD should display the speaker and their slides simultaneously. The accompanying handouts are usually available on a CD or hard copy to follow along. The CDs are great means of reinforcement for those who have a commute or are a nice accompaniment during exercise.

In summary, a review course (or courses) is a useful tool in your armamentarium of resources. The easiest and most helpful report card can be obtained from trusted colleagues who have attended courses previously. However, do your homework to determine which course(s) best fulfills your needs.

## Tutorial Courses

A number of companies and review courses offer instruction and mentoring specific to the oral exam. These courses, if provided as an additional service of the review course, are a separate and distinct service. They differ in that their focus is on strategy, whereas the review course focus is on content.

You should carefully evaluate what each tutorial service has to offer, just as you would for your review course. These tutorial courses typically last one to three days. They usually refer to themselves as a workshop, seminar, or symposium to distinguish them from a review course. Ideally, you want the size limited to no more than 20 to 30 people to ensure you will receive personal attention.

The tutorial course should cover what to expect in terms of exam format and content, as well as providing tips on how to conduct yourself during the exam. A tutorial course should outline the format of the exam so you know exactly what to expect when you walk into your exam room. You should be provided with a list of the exam topics and the expected exam focus. The review course should review each topic on the list. For example, a tutorial course will emphasize that shoulder dystocia is a hot topic and that you must know the maneuvers. The review course will *review* the topic shoulder dystocia in general, of which only one component is the various maneuvers.

A tutorial course will coach you in order to specifically prepare you for the oral exam. Tutorials usually offer assistance in case list preparation, including strategic construction and/or how to defend your case list. Finally, you should be coached about the technique of the oral exam. There should be some didactic lectures to educate you on the approach, but especially there should be the opportunity to practice your newfound skills with your cohorts and local/regional colleagues.

However, the icing on the cake for any tutorial course should be utilizing the course faculty. Although you can prepare capably on your own, the course faculty can help you get there by the quickest and straightest route. They should have the inside scoop on exam topics and examiner conduct based upon feedback from previous candidates. Thus, they should have the know-how and experience to put you through your paces and simulate the exam environment. More importantly, they can give you specific tips to enhance your chance of passing your exam. The disadvantage is that a tutorial course represents an additional expense beyond the review course. However, in only a few sessions you can probably address your deficiencies and get guidance regarding how to use your resources back home so you can continue to practice and improve.

There are two ideal times to take a tutorial course. The first is *before* you begin collecting your case list (e.g., late spring or early summer the year before your exam). This approach allows for the best utilization of tips on case list collection. In particular, this strategy avoids the frustration created by choosing the wrong computer program for data entry. One of the most common responses to "What would you do differently?" is "I would have bailed out of the ABOG case list program." Unfortunately, by the time most candidates acknowledge their error, the time spent to reenter the data in a new program equals the time lost in continuing to struggle with the ABOG program.

Very few candidates have the insight or are so proactive to be this organized. Don't fret. Take the workshop when you are about half way into collecting your cases. By this time, you will be familiar with the process and can be more attentive to the strategy rather than the process. If you decide to bail out of the ABOG case list software, you will have plenty of time to switch systems and reenter your data. The bottom line is to get some professional guidance on how to artfully and strategically construct that case list *before* you submit it August 1. You will be so glad you did, as it is so much easier to defend a well constructed case list. After August 1, your case list is set in stone.

The other ideal time to attend a tutorial course is one to two months before your exam. Now you know the exact topics on your case list. The focus is now how to defend it with competence and confidence. The workshop should prepare you with both didactics and with a mock oral exam/case list review.

The tutorial and review courses are not interchangeable; rather they nicely complement each other. If you can only attend one or the other, then definitely attend the review course. However, the ultimate preparation would be to attend *both* a review course and a tutorial workshop.

It is imperative that you research and compare the different tutorial services. How long has the company been around? Who are the faculty, and how long have they been teaching the workshop? Are all the mock oral examiners clinicians? What is the pass rate of prior course attendees? Of course, the best recommendation is from a satisfied customer. A reputable course should readily offer you a list of references from past participants. The tutorial course will allow you to put it all together. Here you find out what stuff you're made of. If you fail to perform adequately, then a good tutorial course will provide you with the tools needed to refine and polish your presentation.

## Milestones

How did the pygmies eat the elephant? One bite at a time! I will give you a plan for *when* and *how big* your bites should be. It is based on the military tool of milestones, which are dates by which each specific task must be completed to accomplish the mission.

Developing the milestones chart is easy. Simply define the mission, determine the time required to complete the individual tasks, back plot the time, and voilà!—this is when you start. Saying it is one thing; doing it is quite another.

**TABLE 1**   Milestones for the Traditional Track

| Time | Task |
| --- | --- |
| Fall (year preceding the exam) | Review course and/or Case List Construction Workshop |
| June (year preceding the exam) | Order previous year's case list software |
| 1 July-30 June | Case list collection |
| September-October | Order current ABOG case list software |
| February | Request application |
| February | Case List Construction Workshop, if not already done |
| 15 March | Application, fee, copy of medical license, and photographs due |
| 16 March-15 April | Late application plus late fee |
| 16 April-30 April | Late application plus additional late fee |
| 30 April | No applications accepted after this date |
| 1 May-1 June | Case List Construction Workshop, if not already done |
| 15 May-1 June | Send case list to critics for construction tips |

| | |
|---|---|
| April-June | Boards review course and/or Case List Construction Workshop, if not already done |
| 30 June | Complete case list collection |
| July | Receive ABOG notification of admissibility to exam and month of exam |
| 1-10 July | Complete first case list draft |
| 10 July | Send first draft to critics |
| 10-28 July | Complete second case list draft |
| 29 July | Medical records notarization<br>Send case list and examination fee by certified mail |
| 3 August | Case list deadline<br>Examination fee deadline<br>Send case list to critics for defense tips |
| 4-14 August | Late examination fee, late case list fee |
| 3-10 August | Break |
| 14 August | No case lists or examination fees accepted |
| 14-21 August | Collect resources<br>Develop study plan |
| Mid August-September | Intense studying, focused on case list<br>Break one day/week |
| September or October | Meet with critics to review case list defense strategy<br>Boards review course and/or Oral Exam Workshop |
| October (if November exam) | Intense studying, focused on exam probability<br>Mock oral exams<br>    Generalist<br>    Maternal/fetal medicine (MFM) specialist<br>    Reproductive endocrinologist<br>    Oncologist |
| October (if December exam) | Intense studying, focused on case list<br>Break one day/week |
| November (if November exam) | Mock oral exams |
| November (if December exam) | Intense studying, focused on exam probability<br>Boards review course and/or Oral Exam Workshop<br>Mock oral exams |
| November (if January exam) | Intense studying, focused on case list<br>Break one day/week |
| December (if December exam) | Mock oral exams |
| December (if January exam) | Intense studying, focused on exam probability<br>Boards review course and/or Oral Exam Workshop<br>Mock oral exams |
| January (if January exam) | Mock oral exams |

**TABLE 2**   Milestones for the Fast Track

| Time | Task |
|------|------|
| Last Monday in June | Written Board Exam |
| 1 July-30 June | Case list collection |
| June (year preceding the exam) | Order previous year's case list software |
| 1 July-30 June | Case list collection |
| 1 August (year preceding the exam) | Notification of pass/fail on written exam |
| 2 August | Automated application for oral exam and application fee due |
| 12 September | No applications accepted after this date |
| September-October | Order current ABOG case list software |
| 1 October | Notification if accepted into accelerated process |
| 15 May-1 June | Send case list to critics for construction tips |
| April-June | Boards review course and/or Case List Construction Workshop, if not already done |
| 30 June | Complete case list collection |
| July | Receive ABOG notification of admissibility to exam and month of exam |
| 1-10 July | Complete first case list draft |
| 10 July | Send first draft to critics |
| 10-28 July | Complete second case list draft |
| 29 July | Medical records notarization<br>Send case list and examination fee by certified mail |
| 3 August | Case list deadline<br>Examination fee deadline<br>Send case list to critics for defense tips |
| 4-14 August | Late examination fee, late case list fee |
| 3-10 August | Break |
| 14 August | No case lists or examination fees accepted |
| 14–21 August | Collect resources<br>Develop study plan |
| Mid August-September | Intense studying, focused on case list<br>Break one day/week |
| September or October | Meet with critics to review case list defense strategy<br>Boards review course and/or Oral Exam Workshop |
| October (if November exam) | Intense studying, focused on exam probability<br>Mock oral exams<br>    Generalist<br>    Maternal/fetal medicine (MFM) specialist<br>    Reproductive endocrinologist<br>    Oncologist |

| | |
|---|---|
| October (if December exam) | Intense studying, focused on case list<br>Break one day/week |
| November (if November exam) | Mock oral exams |
| November (if December exam) | Intense studying, focused on exam probability<br>Boards review course and/or Oral Exam Workshop<br>Mock oral exams |
| November (if January exam) | Intense studying, focused on case list<br>Break one day/week |
| December (if December exam) | Mock oral exams |
| December (if January exam) | Intense studying, focused on exam probability<br>Boards review course and/or Oral Exam Workshop<br>Mock oral exams |
| January (if January exam) | Mock oral exams |

**TABLE 3**    Milestones for the Fast Track for Fellows

| Time | Task |
|---|---|
| Last Monday in June | Written Board Exam for incoming fellows |
| 1 July of $1^{st}$, $2^{nd}$, $3^{rd}$, or $4^{th}$ | Begin case list collection fellowship year |
| June (year preceding the exam) | Order previous year's case list software |
| 1 August (year preceding the exam) | Notification of pass/fail on written exam |
| 2 August | Automated application for oral exam and application fee due |
| 12 September | No applications accepted after this date |
| September-October | Order current ABOG case list software |
| 1 October | Notification if accepted into accelerated process |
| 15 May-1 June | Send case list to critics for construction tips |
| April-June | Boards review course and/or Case list Construction Workshop, if not already done |
| 30 June | Complete case list collection |
| July | Receive ABOG notification of admissibility to exam and month of exam |
| 1-10 July | Complete first case list draft |
| 10 July | Send first draft to critics |
| 10-28 July | Complete second case list draft |
| 29 July | Medical records notarization<br>Send case list and examination fee by certified mail |
| 3 August | Case list deadline<br>Examination fee deadline<br>Send case list to critics for defense tips |

| | |
|---|---|
| 4-14 August | Late examination fee, late case list fee |
| 3-10 August | Break |
| 14 August | No case lists or examination fees accepted |
| 14-21 August | Collect resources<br>Develop study plan |
| Mid August-September | Intense studying, focused on case list<br>Break one day/week |
| September or October | Meet with critics to review case list defense strategy<br>Boards review course and/or Oral Exam Workshop |
| October (if November exam) | Intense studying, focused on exam probability<br>Mock oral exams<br>    Generalist<br>    Maternal/fetal medicine (MFM) specialist<br>    Reproductive endocrinologist<br>    Oncologist |
| October (if December exam) | Intense studying, focused on case list<br>Break one day/week |
| November (if November exam) | Mock oral exams |
| November (if December exam) | Intense studying, focused on exam probability<br>Boards review course and/or Oral Exam Workshop<br>Mock oral exams |
| November (if January exam) | Intense studying, focused on case list<br>Break one day/week |
| December (if December exam) | Mock oral exams |
| December (if January exam) | Intense studying, focused on exam probability<br>Boards review course and/or Oral Exam Workshop<br>Mock oral exams |
| January (if January exam) | Mock oral exams |

Tables 1, 2 and 3 summarize the milestones for the traditional and fast tracks, respectively. The estimate of the time required for each step will vary with each person. Candid, realistic soul-searching must be employed to analyze how best to modify the milestones for you. Periodically review the timetable, and adjust it accordingly to accomplish the end goal.

The secret for success with the milestone system is timing. Timing is the art of synchronizing events resulting in the optimal outcome—in other words, when all the pieces of the puzzle fall into place. Timing is critical in three areas: case list organization, peer review, and the study plan.

Because the time from the end of the case list data collection (June 30) to the deadline for turning it in (August 1) is so tight, you must have a definite plan to act quickly and implement your strategy. I have yet to meet a candidate who was pleased with the original draft of his/her case list. As a matter of fact, one of the most common regrets expressed by previous candidates is that of running out of time to edit their case list. Ideally, you will have been able to take advantage of a case list construction workshop earlier and already have a plan to implement your strategy and are readily familiar with the software to allow prompt editing. The four weeks allotted for organization of the case list allows time for only one rewrite.

The first draft of the completed case list should be accomplished by mid-July. To meet this deadline, the recommendations from your reviewers must be received no later than July 1. Obviously, you must give them their respective sections in time to accommodate their schedule.

With approximately four weeks remaining, most candidates usually have time for only one rewrite. Again you are at the mercy of your reviewer's schedule to incorporate the second set of recommendations. Apologetically make clear the deadline, emphasizing that you will need that time to incorporate their suggestions. Make your edits as soon as each becomes available rather than when the entire case list is done, to avoid running out of time.

Since half the exam is based on defending your case list, the initial time spent on strategic organization will be much appreciated when you plan your defense. This is your only chance to influence the examiner's first impression, since he or she receives the case list before the first handshake on the day of the exam. This is the first time that many candidates have begun to think seriously about preparing for the exam; clearly, those who charge into battle well prepared on July 1 have the edge.

The second critical milestone category is peer review. Critique of your case list, as well as mock oral exams, is invaluable. Reviewers will see the obvious that you outright missed. The first opportunity for case list review is when your compilation is nearing the end. Send the obstetrics section to your referring maternal-fetal medicine specialist and/or a local generalist. Send the gynecologic section to your oncologist and/or generalist, and send the office practice section to your reproductive endocrinologist or generalist. The specialist more than likely will reflect the profile of the examiner, but the local generalist will be more familiar with your mode of practice. For a professional opinion, attend one of the review courses or tutorial courses that can provide seasoned faculty, experienced in reviewing case lists, to troubleshoot your case list and offer savvy tips on construction.

Allow ample time for review, but also be up front about your deadline. Send the first batch in May or June, and set a due date of July 1. Send the next draft back to the reviewer by mid-July with a due date in the third week of July. The purpose of this peer review from May through July is to make recommendations for the strategic organization and construction of the case list. Send your masterpiece back in August and/or September. The goal then is to help plan its defense. You may again want a pair of professional eyes to identify expected questions and especially ideal answers for your exam.

The ultimate test of the depth and breadth of your knowledge (and your ability to convey that knowledge) is the mock oral exam. Because most of us are unfamiliar with oral examinations and hence intimidated by that format, there is a natural tendency to procrastinate or, worse yet, to avoid this valuable study tool. Most physicians are stereotypically their own worst critics. They underestimate their abilities and delay a mock oral to study even more, hoping to avoid the embarrassing acknowledgment that they don't know everything. This tactic is self-defeating because your peers and the examiners already know that you can't possibly know it all.

I recommend a planning session for case list defense strategy in September. Meet with each of the colleagues to whom you sent the sections for case list organization tips. Most valuable of all is to schedule a mock oral exam with each colleague the month before your exam. The final test is a mock oral exam with a peer(s) who is unfamiliar to you (such as the review or tutorial course faculty member). Again, a mock oral exam may be better left to the professionals whose recommendations are based on years of feedback with their tried and true tips.

After the case list is set in stone, the final major milestone is to determine *what* you need to study and *when*. The *what* process is outlined in Chapter 8: Studying for the Exam. Recall that study topics are prioritized by exam probability: topics likely to appear because of their occurrence on previous exams and topics generated by your case list. The prioritizing of these topics is based on your comfort with your knowledge base for each topic.

Determining when or, more specifically, how long to devote to each study topic is an art learned only through experience. It is gained only upon realizing that studying for the oral boards is completely different from studying for the written boards. To study for the orals in the same manner as for the written boards is a waste of precious time. A written exam by nature is restricted to individual questions within a specific topic.

The oral exam is an evaluation of your collective understanding of the topic and your ability to apply that knowledge to patient management. Thus, studying for the oral exam should be limited to a comprehensive, clinically oriented review—not an exhaustive, in-depth understanding laden with textbook facts.

Incredible discipline is required to restrict your study to a review. Tackling the first few topics is all that is necessary to learn the new focus and to gain an appreciation of the time required to cover a topic. After you get the hang of it, go back and revise your original study timetable accordingly.

In conclusion, timing is everything. The oral exam is clearly an example of the proverb, "Forewarned is forearmed." Undoubtedly, anyone who has passed the written board exam is academically capable of passing his or her oral boards. But those who methodically and diligently stick to their plan will accomplish this feat much more easily.

**Chapter**

# The Case List

## Significance of the Exam

The ABOG *Bulletin* states that half of your exam is defending your case list. The case list is a far more accurate assessment of your mode of practice than a mere three hours of testing. It is a year-long culmination of applying book knowledge to clinical practice. Furthermore, a candidate's mode of practice continues to be the number-one reason for failing the oral board exam. Thus, in my opinion, the single most important component of the oral examination is the case list.

The examiners receive your case list at least the day prior to your exam. Certainly, the degree of scrutiny varies with each examiner and the number of lists he receives. Nevertheless, the examiner meets your case list before he meets you. Undoubtedly, he will form a first impression of you based exclusively on your case list.

I have reviewed many case lists. Outright failures, although rare, are obvious. On the other hand, there are no guaranteed passes based on the case list alone. The other test components (e.g., case of the day) and especially your finesse with the oral exam format greatly influence the outcome. However, as long as you do not outright flunk the other exam components, you will surely pass the exam if you have satisfactorily defended your case list.

Thus, sound performance on the oral exam and a solid case list defense are a sure bet for passing. An unsound case list, regardless of a stellar performance on the exam, will most likely result in failure. An unsound case list and a weak performance on the exam are guaranteed to result in failure.

## Criteria for Admission to the Exam

The case list is a compilation of office and hospital patients for whom you personally provided care during the 12 months preceding June 30 of the year of your exam. This implies that you (not your partner or residents) personally controlled the medical and/or surgical management of each patient listed. You cannot reuse any case or case list from a previous examination. If you are a generalist, you must submit a case list in all three areas. If your practice is limited to obstetrics *or* gynecology, you must submit a case list in your area of specialty, and a minimum of 20 selected patients from your chief year in the other area. Regardless, you will be examined in *all three areas*: obstetrics, gynecology, and office practice.

All candidates must have an office and a hospital practice. The case list must include 40 office practice patients *and* a minimum of 20 hospitalized and/or ambulatory gynecologic *and* 20 hospitalized obstetric patients with significant problems.

If the minimum of 20 obstetrical and 20 gynecological hospital-based patients cannot be obtained within the one-year deadline, then you have two options. You can submit an additional *complete* six-month case list of the patients managed immediately prior to the 12-month period, namely January 1 to June 30, or you can submit patients from your chief year of residency to complete the list of 20 gynecological and/or 20 obstetrical cases. You cannot submit a case list comprised solely of cases from your chief year. Thus, you will then submit two lists, with a minimum of 40 hospitalized patients for 12 months' duration and one of six months' duration, and/or a case list from your chief year.

Case lists for subspecialists must meet the same criteria discussed above for those practitioners with a limited practice. In other words, your case list must contain obstetrical and gynecological cases either from your practice and/or from your fellowship or chief residency log. If you are still in your fellowship training, then you can sit for your general boards only once in your fellowship and no earlier than your second year. Furthermore, you cannot sit for your subspecialty boards until you pass your general boards.

If this is as clear as mud, I suggest you check with the ABOG *Bulletin* or write ABOG for clarification. I want to emphasize that **all** candidates will be tested in **all three** areas of obstetrics, gynecology, and office practice.

## Collection of the Case List

No other phase of preparation for the exam requires as much discipline as the collection of the case list. Since it is a year-long compilation, there is a tendency to procrastinate. Not surprisingly, however, procrastination creates a domino effect—last-minute scrambling and haste that truly makes waste. Precious details are best recalled when fresh.

There are three sections to the case list: obstetrics, gynecology, and office practice. ABOG provides the forms with the specific format for recording each section (see Appendix D). Every gynecologic surgery and hospitalized obstetric patient must be logged, whereas only 40 patients from the 40 office practice categories are necessary.

Recall from Chapter 2: The Application Process that you cannot formally request an application until February of the year of your exam. Yet the time frame that the case list covers started was way back in July 1. To delay until February would result in a dangerous, self-perpetuating backlog because ongoing data continue to accrue.

To avoid always being behind the eight ball, I recommend that you obtain the preceding year's forms by July 1. The only risk is that the form format may change (but they haven't in years), necessitating a reentry of data. The benefit of timely data collection far outweighs the unlikely risk of having to transfer data to revised forms.

How often you should update your case list is highly variable. Feedback from previous candidates reveals the average time is weekly. In my opinion, the ideal time is immediately after every patient, when recall is at its peak. The least frequent update, without risking significantly compromised recall, is bimonthly.

The method of recording the data depends on individual preference. In any case, the initial log should be readily transportable. Unless you have a personal computer (PC or Mac) or a Palm Pilot or another PDA (personal digital assistant) that you can readily lug around, the best initial means is still paper. Carry blank copies of the obstetric and gynecologic ABOG forms, and complete the form immediately after every delivery or surgery.

The office practice case list collection is no less challenging just because it is only 40 patients. Although it is certainly not necessary to begin collecting these patients on July 1, there is a tendency to procrastinate and all of a sudden be behind. Additionally, you must put some thought into which of the 40 categories you want to select. Remember, you don't have a choice on the obstetrics or gynecology list. Keep the list of the 40 categories on your desk. Add the names of the representative patients no later than January.

Common office practice categories, such as menopause, vaginitis, and preventive care, will fill up quickly. Since a maximum of two patients can be listed in each category, it is not necessary to collect more than four patients. Uncommon categories, such as pediatric gynecology and rape, may take months, if at all, to find. The collection of patients in rare categories is obviously most compromised by procrastination.

Your first rough draft needs to be edited and entered in accordance with the ABOG requirements. You may either submit the data to your transcriptionist or enter them yourself. There are pros and cons for each option. Do not waste time if you are unfamiliar or unskilled with either. Be efficient with revisions; make them purposeful and strategic. Knowing what to edit is usually not obvious until the entire case list is entered. Since data compilation ends June 30 and the case list is due August 1, little time remains for more than one major revision.

You can save time by having someone else enter your data on the ABOG forms. This option allows you to "step away" from that task and tackle the revisions later. You must, however, make your intention crystal-clear to avoid losing time in correcting miscommunications. The most obvious disadvantage is that you are dependent on someone else's schedule. Make it clear that the clock is ticking, and give specific deadlines. Remember also that procrastination on your part does not justify an emergency on theirs.

You can avoid these hassles by entering the data yourself. ABOG offers a computer software program. Because it is endorsed by ABOG, many candidates erroneously assume that it is the only acceptable program. This is not true. Any program may be used as long as it complies with the specific ABOG format.

The ABOG program has some bugs, generates frustration, and wastes time. Feedback from candidates who have tried both the ABOG program and their own program is overwhelmingly in favor of their own. Thus, if you choose to use the computer as a vehicle for data entry, I recommend use of your own program. Tips on how to do so (and on how to use the ABOG program) are found in Appendix D. Choose the program that seems to you the easiest and most adaptable to editing.

Finally, you must personally tally your summary sheets by hand. The ABOG program and often even customized programs do not count correctly.

I recommend that you have several checks and balances to make sure that your tally is accurate. Keep a log of every hospitalized obstetric and gynecologic patient. In addition, create a log based on each of the categories listed in the summary sheet. Include a description of each category if the categories are ambiguous. List the corresponding patient's name, date, and diagnosis or procedure for quick cross-reference. Most importantly, check your numbers—and check them twice.

## Initial Draft: Case-by-Case Entry

The case list will make or break you. Thus, you should painstakingly plan its organization and your defense. Your first opportunity is the initial entry on the ABOG forms. For each patient, draft a narrative summary of the patient management issues as if you were presenting her at morning report or teaching rounds. This clinical summary is the stepping stone from which you will later extract the pertinent data to complete the ABOG forms. Now let's discuss each of the three sections.

## List of Obstetric Patients

List *separately* each patient with a complication or abnormality, along with medical and surgical interventions during pregnancy, labor, delivery, and the puerperium. Although the final copy will list only complicated patients, I recommend that you draft a clinical narrative for every delivery. Sometimes it is not obvious into which category a patient falls until later review.

Ultimately you will simply list a total of the **number** of normal, uncomplicated obstetrical patients on the summary sheet. You will not list these patients individually on your case list as you will for the complicated ones. ABOG defines a normal uncomplicated patient by the following criteria:

A. Pregnancy, labor, delivery, and the puerperium were uncomplicated, and labor began spontaneously between the 37th and 42nd week of gestation;

B. The membranes ruptured or were ruptured after labor began;

C. Presentation was vertex, position occiput anterior or transverse, and labor was less than 24 hours in duration;

D. Delivery was spontaneous or by outlet forceps with or without episiotomy, from an anterior position;

E. The infant had a five-minute Apgar score of 6 or more, weighed between 2500 and 4500 grams, and was healthy; and

F. Uncomplicated delivery of the placenta and blood loss less than 500 ml.

All deliveries not fulfilling these criteria must be listed separately. The total number of deliveries (> 500 grams), both complicated and uncomplicated, are tallied at the end of the obstetric list and on the summary sheet.

A minimum of 20 patients is required on the obstetrics list from the categories listed below. Although you must list *all* complicated patients, you cannot *count* more than *two* patients from each category to meet the minimum requirement of 20 patients. For example, if you have four breech presentations, you must report all four on your case list, but only two of the four will be counted as meeting the minimum requirement of 20 cases.

## *Obstetrical Categories*

1. Abnormal fetal growth
2. Any maternal complication that delayed hospital discharge by 48 or more hours
3. Any neonatal complication that delayed hospital discharge by 48 or more hours
4. Breech and other fetal malpresentations
5. Cardiovascular and/or pulmonary diseases complicating pregnancy
6. Cesarean hysterectomy
7. Hematologic diseases and/or endocrine diseases complicating pregnancy
8. Hypertensive disorders of pregnancy (chronic hypertension, preeclampsia, eclampsia)
9. Inductions and/or augmentations of labor
10. Infections complicating pregnancy
11. Intrapartum infection (amnionitis)
12. Multifetal pregnancy
*13. *Obstetrical vaginal lacerations ($3^{rd}$ and $4^{th}$ degree lacerations)*
14. Post-term pregnancy

*15. *Preconception evaluation, prenatal, and genetic diagnoses*

16. Pregnancies complicated by human immunodeficiency virus (HIV) infection

*17. *Pregnancies and coexisting malignancies*

18. Premature rupture of membranes at term (PROM)

19. Preterm delivery

20. Preterm premature rupture of membranes (PPROM)

21. Pregnancies complicated by fetal anomalies

22. Primary Cesarean delivery

23. Puerperal hemorrhage

24. Puerperal infection

25. Readmission for maternal complications up to 6 weeks post partum

26. Renal diseases and/or neurologic diseases complicating pregnancy

27. Repeat Cesarean delivery

28. Second-trimester spontaneous abortion

29. Third-trimester bleeding

*30. *Trauma in pregnancy (automobile accidents)*

31. Vaginal birth after cesarean delivery (VBAC)

32. All other cases

 * Recent new categories

Whereas each complicated obstetric patient is listed, only the total number of normal, uncomplicated obstetric patients is tallied on the summary sheet. To ensure listing only appropriate patients, initially complete the ABOG form **for all** deliveries. You can later delete the uncomplicated patients after you are certain they are indeed a normal delivery.

The summary sheet should be hand tallied. Record **all** the patients that you managed in each category in the "total cases" column. This reflects your depth of experience in each category. Recall, however, that you can apply only two patients from each category to count toward your mandatory minimum of 20 patients. These are recorded on the "total applied" column. The sum of the total applied is placed in the "total cases" and obviously must be 20 or more. The total number of deliveries will be the sum of the "total cases" and "total uncomplicated spontaneous deliveries" categories.

"OB ultrasounds and color Doppler examinations" is the number of ultrasounds performed by *you* on hospitalized obstetrical patients. Note again that this is the number that you personally performed, not those that you ordered and were performed by a technician or radiologist.

The Cesarean Delivery (CD) categories on the summary sheet do not necessarily represent your Cesarean delivery rate. Although a patient may have indeed had a CD, she may be applied to a different category. For example, if you performed a CD for a patient with a breech presentation, you may list her in either the "breech and other fetal malpresentations" or "Cesarean Delivery" category, but not both. Even though the summary sheet no longer has a category for overall number of CDs, **you must** know your primary, repeat, and total CD rate. If you are asked, you will have a ready answer, as it is surely not a good time to get your calculator out in the middle of your exam.

The number of other obstetrical considerations is the final category of the summary sheet. This consists of "Apgar ≤5, infants < 2,500 grams, and perinatal deaths." Each of these categories also show in separate headings in the columns of the obstetric list. Thus, it is easy for the examiner to cross reference these from the summary sheet to the case list by quickly searching out the outliers in their respective columns.

ABOG's only guidance on what to include on the entry sheet is the column headings. Don't misinterpret the antepartum complications column as only labor issues. This column should also include complications that occurred throughout the prenatal course. If you list only labor issues, the examiner has a free rein to come up with any hypothetical prenatal topic of his choice. Common sense should prevail; challenges in patient care don't start with the first contraction, but rather from the time of conception.

Although the content of the columns varies in subjectivity, understand what each column represents. Column confusion is the *most common mistake* in constructing the obstetric case list. The columns most often confused are *Complications of Antepartum, Complications of Delivery or Postpartum*, and *Operative Procedures and/or Treatment*. Include only the information that applies to that specific column. The confusion is due to differing interpretations when distinguishing antepartum from delivery. When does antepartum end and delivery begin?

Unfortunately, the customary division of labor into three stages does not fully clarify the debate. The first stage of labor begins with the onset of uterine contractions sufficient to efface the cervix and ends with complete cervical dilatation. The second stage of labor begins with complete cervical dilatation and ends with the expulsion of the infant. The third stage of labor is the separation and expulsion of the placenta.

Thus, the *Antepartum* column clearly includes complications of pregnancy and the first stage of labor. Likewise, the *Delivery or Postpartum* column includes any complications of the third stage of labor up to 6 weeks postpartum. In which column do stage two complications belong? Does delivery include all of stage two, including pushing? Or is delivery purely the actual extraction or expulsion of the fetus? You can make an argument to include stage two complications in either the *Antepartum* or the *Delivery or Postpartum* column. Whichever you choose, be consistent throughout the case list.

I recommend that any complications up to and including complete cervical dilatation be listed in the *Antepartum* column. This includes disorders of protracted dilatation and arrest of dilatation. Any complication thereafter—namely, arrest of descent, instrumented deliveries, and shoulder dystocias—can be listed in either the *Antepartum* or *Delivery or Postpartum* column. Table 1 summarizes recommended listings for common complications as well as possible treatment options.

**TABLE 1** Recommended Listings and Treatment Options for Common Complications

| Complication | Antepartum | Delivery or Postpartum | Operative Procedure and/or Treatment |
|---|---|---|---|
| Protracted labor | X | | Pitocin augmentation |
| Arrest of dilatation | X | | Pitocin augmentation and/or CD |
| Arrest of descent | X | X | Vacuum/forceps or CD |
| Cephalopelvic disproportion | X | X | Cesarean delivery |
| Shoulder dystocia | | X | List of maneuvers optional |
| Retained placenta | | X | Manual extraction |
| Uterine atony | | X | Uterotonic agent |

Example 1 (page 75) shows how the complications of protracted labor and non-reassuring FHR were listed in the wrong column. They should be listed in the *Complications of Antepartum* column, not in the *Complications of Delivery and Postpartum* column. I hope to convince you later, in the

"Strategic organization of the case list" section of this chapter, that your column selection reflects your logical and chronological thought process of patient management.

Be reasonable in your interpretation of a complication. I interpret a complication as any event or issue that *significantly* influences your management. You do not want to bog down your case list with copious insignificant data. For example, I would not list a patient if the only issue in an otherwise uncomplicated pregnancy, labor, and delivery was advanced maternal age. On the other hand, if the patient became preeclamptic or carried a fetus with a trisomy, advanced maternal age might be listed as a complication (although you have to list the patient's age in any case). Similarly, I would not list a patient who had an abnormal quadruple screen if further testing was normal. I would list her only if further testing was persistently abnormal without an identifiable cause or if she carried a fetus with a neural tube defect. A simple rule of thumb is to decide whether you would present the patient in your morning report or changeover. If the answer is yes, list her; otherwise, count her as normal and uncomplicated.

How you word a problem greatly influences its interpretation and defense. If it's best to call a rose a rose, then do so. This is especially true if you have only one representative case. In other words, if you have only one gestational diabetic, then be specific in her management in the procedures and/or treatment column. On the other hand, if you have a number of diabetics, then you can word the majority's treatment as "routine diabetic care."

If you choose to be generic, however, you must have a sprinkling of the specifics so that the examiner can deduce what you mean by routine care. For the most part, make it evident how you manage diabetics. If he wants further details, then he can ask you. However, if you worded the treatment for all your patients with the same problem without specific details, then it is unknown how you manage such patients. This is risky, for if the examiner does not get time to validate the specifics, then he is forced to assume you don't know. Like the medical chart, if it's not documented, it didn't happen.

The columns that dictate objective data are straightforward: *Patient #, Hospital #, Age, Gravida, Days in Hospital, Perinatal Death, Newborn Weight,* and *Apgar*. Initially, include the patient's name to aid in your recall of the case. But absolutely, your final copy must de-identify her in order to be compliant with the Health Insurance Portability and Accounting Act of 1996 (HIPAA). Effective 2008, ABOG allows you to bring your case list that you intend to use for the exam with the patient's initials.

The # refers to the sequential ordering **for all** patients from all hospitals, so every patient will have a unique number. This is what the examiner refers to when he says, "Tell me about patient # ___." The *hospital* # refers to the sequential ordering of hospitals being reported from. For example, if you admit patients to two hospitals, then you will list the hospitals as Hospital A and B, respectively. The *patient* # refers to the sequential ordering of patients reported from a given hospital. Let's say you deliver two patients from two different hospitals. The first is #1, and her *hospital* # is "A" and her *patient* # is "A-1," whereas the second patient is #2, and her *hospital* # is "B" and her *patient* # is "B-1."

*Parity* means just that; do not enumerate further with abortions, preterm delivery, living offspring, or ectopic pregnancies. List the *Gestational Age* at admission and round off in whole numbers, not fractions (e.g., 41 weeks, not 41-2/7 or 41+).

The *days in the hospital* are the number of days, and not the dates. The newborn's *weight* is reported in grams.

Effective in 2008 you must check at the top of each case list page, whether the source of each case was from *post-residency cases, senior residency cases* or *fellowship cases.* Traditionally, it was not as obvious that a case list belonged to a subspecialist unless there were exactly 20 patients. However, now it's flashing in marquee lights at the top of each page. I doubt this engenders any mercy for the candidate defending his non-specialty or, on the other hand, to be more scrutinized in the specialty area. The criteria for pass/fail should be the same for all. Note, however, that the examiners tend to be subspecialists.

Be precise in terminology, especially for dysfunction of labor. At a minimum, use the appropriate Friedman terminology (Table 2) to justify augmentation of labor and cesarean sections. Certainly, the duration threshold originally proposed for labor dysfunction, especially in the setting of an epidural, have come under fire recently. The key is to avoid the diagnosis "failure to progress" because it is vague and does not convey an understanding of the pathophysiology of labor. Make sure that your procedure and treatment are substantiated by the indicating complication.

I remind you again, it is imperative that you submit a de-identified case list to ABOG. Failure to do so will result in your case list being summarily rejected. Not only do you not get to pass go, but you also do not collect $200. You do, however, get to collect a whole new case list for next year!

**TABLE 2** Abnormal Labor Patterns, Diagnostic Criteria, and Methods of Treatment

| Labor Pattern | Diagnostic Criteria | | Preferred Treatment | Exceptional Treatment |
| --- | --- | --- | --- | --- |
| | Nulligravidas | Multiparas | | |
| Prolongation disorder<br>1. Prolonged latent phase | >20hr | >14hr | Therapeutic rest | Oxytocin or cesarean sections for urgent problems |
| Protraction disorders<br>1. Protracted active phase dialation | <1.2cm/hr | <1.5cm/hr | | |
| 2. Protracted descent | <1.0cm/hr | <2cm/hr | Expectant and supportive | Cesarean section for CPD |
| Arrest disorders<br>1. Prolonged deceleration phase | >3hr | >1hr | Without CPD: oxytocin | Rest if exhausted |
| 2. Secondary arrest of dilation | >2hr | >2hr | | |
| 3. Arrest of descent | >1hr | >1hr | With CPD: oxytocin | Cesarean section |
| 4. Failure of descent | No descent in deceleration phase or second stage of labor | | | |

CPD = cephalopelvic disproportion.
Modified from Cohen and Friedman, 1983.

Let's tie together all of the above suggestions for initial case entry by an example.

## Clinical Summary

Karen Burke is a 34-year-old 2G/0P/1Ab at 38 weeks EGA. Karen had pre-pregnancy hypertension that had not required medication. As the pregnancy progressed, she developed superimposed preeclampsia and required Aldomet.

At her 38-week office visit, her blood pressure was 160/110, with a five-pound weight gain since the previous week, and 2+ protein. She also complained of a severe headache.

She was sent to Labor and Delivery. Her cervix was unripe, with a Bishop score of 3; therefore, she first underwent successful cervical ripening with prostaglandin E gel. Pitocin induction was initiated, and she progressed to active labor but failed to dilate beyond 5 cm after two hours. An intrauterine pressure catheter was placed and demonstrated adequate Montevideo units, thereby confirming arrest of the active phase of labor. She was delivered by primary cesarean section. The infant weighed 3435 grams and had Apgar scores of 9 and 10.

## Initial ABOG Form Entry

First of all, start a binder for each of the three sections: obstetrics, gynecology, and office practice. Let's start with obstetrics. For each obstetrical patient, insert the clinical summary and the first draft of the ABOG form (see Example 2 on page 75). Ideally, include a copy of her prenatal record and the delivery note. If the patient was particularly complicated, you can supplement further with pertinent copies of other medical records, such as consultations, laboratory, ultrasound reports, etc. Later you will add supporting resources and case list edits.

Begin a handwritten log of the statistics required by the Summary Sheet. Do not rely on the computer for accuracy. Many programs are fraught with inaccurate tallying.

Okay, by this point at least we're out of the starting block. Don't get hung up on the logistics and the nitty-gritty detail. That will come later. As a matter of fact, forget the doggone software if it's confusing and precluding you from starting. Remember the ol' paper and pen?

Just use your common sense to enter the cases on the case list form. I promise you, once you get the hang of it, and it won't take long, you'll be primed to move to the next step. Remember long ago when you were an intern on labor and delivery? The first step was just in learning how to do a cervical check. This is no different.

### List of Gynecologic Patients

All patients who underwent a gynecologic surgical procedure outside the office setting and all non-surgical admissions are listed. The total number of ultrasounds that you personally performed on hospitalized gynecologic patients must also be included, as well as the number of hospital stays more than 7 days.

A minimum of 20 gynecologic patients is required. Although you enter the total number of procedures performed in the "total cases" column, you may count only two patients from each of the categories listed below.

## *Gynecological Categories*

1. Abdominal hysterectomy
*2. *Abnormal cervical cytology* and colposcopy
3. Abnormal uterine bleeding
4. Adenomyosis
5. Adnexal problems excluding ectopic pregnancy and pelvic inflammatory disease
6. Carcinoma *in situ*
7. Congenital abnormalities of the reproductive tract
8. Defects in pelvic floor
9. Diagnostic laparoscopy
10. Ectopic pregnancy
11. Endometriosis
12. Invasive carcinoma
13. Laparotomy (other than tubal sterilization) infertility evaluation
14. Operative hysteroscopy infertility treatment
15. Operative laparoscopy (other than tubal sterilization)
*16. *Operative management of* pelvic pain
17. Pelvic inflammatory disease
18. Postoperative fever for greater than 48 hours
19. Postoperative throbophlebitis and/or embolism
20. Postoperative wound complications
*21. *Preoperative evaluation of coexisting conditions (respiratory, cardiac, metabolic diseases)*
22. Rectovaginal or urinary tract fistula
23. Tubal sterilization
24. Urinary *and fecal* incontinence (*operative management*)
*25. *Urinary incontinence (medical management)*
26. Uterine myomas
27. Vaginal hysterectomy (including laparoscopically assisted)
28. Vulvar masses
29. Vulvar ulcers
30. All other cases

\* Recent new categories

The "total applied" column in the Gynecologic Summary sheet cannot have more than two, and the "total cases" of "total applied" must be at least 20. The "total cases" reflects how busy you are. The examiner can quickly determine a profile of the type of surgeon you are by simply perusing the number of cases of each category. The number of hospital stays that exceed seven days is an indicator of how safe a surgeon you are. The examiner can quickly search the column within your case list and confirm his hunches.

As noted for the obstetrics list, understand what each column in the gynecologic form represents and complete each accordingly. The *pre-operative or admission diagnosis* typically supports the treatment. The pre-operative diagnosis should include pertinent non-surgical as well as conservative surgical therapy. For example, the pre-operative diagnosis of menometrorrhagia could be further qualified by lack of response to hormonal therapy or a D&C.

As discussed in the obstetrics list, how you word a problem greatly influences interpretation and defense. I remind you that if it is best to call a rose a rose, then do so. However, if you chose to be generic, then you must have a sprinkling of the specifics so that the examiner can deduce what you mean by routine care. Using the above example of menometrorrhagia, on some scattered patients, you might list specific treatment of progesterone, OCPs, IUD, DMPA, or GnRH agonists. For the most part, it's clear by what you mean by hormonal or medical therapy. If he wants further details, then he can ask you. However, if you worded the treatment for all your patients with the same problem generically, then it is unknown how you manage such patients. This is risky, for if the examiner does not get time to validate the specifics, then he is forced to assume that you don't know.

We'll talk later about how to handle the situation when you performed two separate operations on the same patient within the same year (e.g., both a D&C and then later a hysterectomy). For non-surgical conditions, the admission diagnosis is listed in the preoperative diagnosis column too.

You want to make it clear in the preoperative diagnosis column why you took the patient to the operating room and that the procedure performed was appropriate. If you simply list "ovarian cyst" as the preoperative diagnosis, then the examiner doesn't know if it was appropriate to have performed a laparoscopy. The size of ovarian cysts must be recorded in centimeters in the preoperative diagnosis. Although not mandatory, I strongly recommend you further qualify the cyst by type (simple or complex), side (left, right, or bilateral) and tumor markers, if appropriate.

Likewise, you want to list a stage or grade for prolapse cases. If you simply list uterine prolapse, then how does the examiner know that the procedure performed was appropriate or overkill? Clearly, the preoperative diagnosis of procidentia warrants support of the apex, so "vaginal hysterectomy" isn't sufficient. On the other hand, "VH with uterosacral suspension, TVT" satisfies the examiner's concerns that the apex was well supported and that prophylactic support of the urethra will avoid post-op urinary incontinence.

The *treatment* column should include all surgical procedures. It should also include primary non-surgical treatment if the patient was admitted but not operated on. For example, your *preoperative or admission diagnosis* is PID and your *treatment* is pareneteral antibiotics. Non-primary treatment should be listed in the preoperative or admission diagnosis column. Let's say this patient did not respond to antibiotics and you had to take her to the OR. In this setting your *preoperative or admission diagnosis* may state "PID, tubo-ovarian abscess refractory to antibiotics," and the *treatment* may be "exploratory laparotomy, lysis of adhesions, drainage of tubo-ovarian abscess".

The pathologic diagnosis should support the preoperative diagnosis. For example, if the preoperative diagnosis is menometrorrhagia secondary to leiomyomata, the pathology should verify a leiomyomatous uterus. Furthermore, include only the pertinent pathology, not the entire pathology report, and list the offending organ first. In this example, list first the uterus, the weight in grams and simply list: leiomyomata, and cervix benign.

Hysterectomy specimens must include the uterine weight in grams. In cases without tissue for histologic diagnosis, the final clinical diagnosis should be listed. For example, let's say your preoperative diagnosis is "chronic pelvic pain refractory to conservative measures." Your treatment is "operative laparoscopy," but you didn't remove any tissue. Thus, you would report your clinical diagnosis, such as "endometriotic implants, dense pelvic adhesions" in the *surgical pathology diagnosis* column.

The *complications* column is subject to interpretation. You must list obvious significant complications, like a ureteral or bowel injury, and you must include blood transfusions. However, some strategic thought must go into just how much detail you feel is appropriate. Again, I wouldn't clutter your case list with insignificant events that didn't change the patient's outcome or hospital stay, so the fact that the patient spiked a fever the evening of surgery but was afebrile within 24 hours is probably irrelevant.

However, if the fever occurred on POD #2 and you had to launch a workup and start parenteral antibiotics, then the details should be included in the *complications* column.

Don't be afraid of the *complications* column. If you operate frequently enough, then you are going to have some complications, just hopefully not on every patient. However, it looks suspicious and deceptive if a case list is *devoid* of *any* complications. Don't even think of selectively (oops) withholding that nightmare complication, such as a death. ABOG does audit, and if you committed fraud, not only do you sit out of your exam for three years, but you must report this disciplinary action for *the rest of your career*!

As in the obstetrics list, The "#" refers to the sequential ordering for **all** patients from all hospitals, so every patient will have a unique number. This is what the examiner means when he says, "Tell me about patient # __." The *hospital #* refers to the sequential ordering of hospitals being reported from. For example, if you admit patients to two hospitals, then you will list them as Hospital A and B, respectively. The *patient #* refers to the sequential ordering of patients reported from a given hospital. So let's say you operate on two patients at two different hospitals. The first is #1, and her *hospital #* is "A" and her *patient #* is "A-1," whereas the second patient is #2, and her *hospital #* is "B" and her *patient #* is "B-1."

Like the obstetrics list, indicate at the top of each case list page, whether the source of each case was from *post-residency cases, senior residency cases,* or *fellowship cases.* The *days in the hospital* is the arithmetic difference between date of discharge and date of admission. So if you did a D&C on an outpatient basis, the patient's number of days in the hospital is zero. If your vaginal hysterectomy patient went home on POD #1, then her number of days in the hospital is one.

Be attentive to details and use precise and up-to-date terminology. For example, use the Bethesda system (SIL) for Pap smear nomenclature rather than CIN. Likewise, the use of "complex" or "simple" alone for endometrial hyperplasia is antiquated and does not influence its management, but the presence or absence of atypia does. The term "fibroid" is acceptable slang but is not as precise or sophisticated as the term "leiomyomata."

As for all the sections, complete the columns with as much information to easily follow your thought process for patient management. You can later trim strategically. To facilitate this process, start once again with a narrative summary of the clinical issues.

## Clinical Summary

Joyce Collins is a 42-year-old 2G/2P who has complained of progressive menorrhagia for the past year. Her menses are monthly and last up to 7 days, whereas previously they lasted only 4-5 days. The second and third days of her periods are so heavy that she is homebound and must change both a simultaneous super tampon and overnight pad every hour while awake. She denies breakthrough bleeding. She has also recently started to experience night sweats. Pelvic exam reveals an 8-10-week size uterus, with several irregular masses consistent with leiomyomata. The ovaries are normal size.

She was initially treated with oral contraceptive pills (OCP). Although her night sweats resolved, she had minimal improvement in menorrhagia after three cycles. She chose conservative surgery and underwent a hysteroscopically guided fractional D&C. She had obvious submucosal leiomyomata, and the secretory pathology was consistent with OCP suppression. The D&C also failed to improve her menorrhagia. Thus, she has elected for definitive therapy. She was counseled on the various routes for hysterectomy, as well as the pros and cons for a prophylactic oophorectomy. She elected for and underwent a vaginal hysterectomy.

## Initial ABOG Form Entry

Joyce Collins presents an uncommon case list quandary in that she had two procedures performed within the same year of case list collections. You can count a patient only once, as each patient must have a unique patient number. You may, however, list both procedures. You can count each procedure in the total cases column of the summary sheet, but can only apply one to a specific category.

See Example 3 on page 76. JC is listed once as #52 and is the only patient with this designator on the gynecology case list. Both the D&C and the vaginal hysterectomy are listed, but each encounter is separated by a deliberate demarcating space between texts. In other words, each encounter should stand alone, such that the preoperative diagnosis supports each treatment.

On the summary sheet, you can assign each procedure to a category. Let's say you put the D&C in the abnormal uterine bleeding category and the vaginal hysterectomy in the vaginal hysterectomy category. However, you can apply only one. It's always advantageous to have as many vaginal hysterectomies as possible, so let's apply her to this category. Thus, the abnormal uterine bleeding category will have one in the total cases column but none for total applied, whereas the vaginal hysterectomy category will have one each in the total cases and total applied columns.

## List of Office Patients

The office practice case list has evolved over the past several years. When the pathology slide section was dropped from the exam in the mid- 1990s, the number of categories in the office practice case list was lengthened. Managed care and CREOG's mandate to push the primary care aspects of obstetrics/gynecology resulted in further additions to the office practice case list.

In 2001, the office list blossomed to 40 categories. Not surprisingly, the new players were in primary care, and the obstetrics-related categories were deleted. Personally performed ultrasounds were also added. To accommodate the longer list of categories, the number of representative patients was expanded from 40 to 60, but in 2004 it was scaled back again to 40. The maximum number of patients in each category was reduced initially from four to three and then again to the current two.

Well, the pendulum is swinging back as OB/GYN practitioners rebelled about being forced into primary care. Most were quite content to remain specialists in women's health. Furthermore, residency training was forced to adapt as well. Since the length of the residency remained unchanged at four years, something had to give to accommodate this additional mandate for primary care training. Unfortunately, the OB and GYN rotations were trimmed. Not surprisingly, these new batches of residents were spread thin and were not as skilled in the specialty. Thus, either the residency had to be lengthened or the primary care requirements loosened. For now, the specialty has won. Thus, all the primary care topics remain, but the heavy emphasis on detail to the level of an internist has been lifted.

Finally, the exam focus is shifting back to what a gynecologist needs to know about primary care issues in order to screen, diagnose, and refer to the internists. Currently, you must list 40 patients. There are now 40 categories, as listed below, but you may list no more than two from any one category.

## *Office Practice Categories*

1. Abnormal uterine bleeding
2. Back pain
3. Benign pelvic masses
4. Breast diseases
5. Cardiovascular diseases
6. Contraception
7. Depression
8. Diagnosis and management of hypercholesterolemia and dyslipidemias
9. Dysmenorrhea
10. Endocrine diseases (diabetes mellitus, thyroid or adrenal disease)
11. Endometriosis
12. Evaluation and Management of Pelvic pain
13. *Evaluation of Urinary and *Rectal* Incontinence
14. Gastrointestinal diseases
15. Genetic counseling
16. Geriatrics
17. Hyperprolactinemia
18. Hypertension
19. Immunizations
20. Infertility
21. *Infertility Evaluation and Management*
22. Office surgery
23. Pediatric gynecology
24. Pelvic floor defects
25. *Perimenopause* and Menopausal Care
26. Premenstrual syndrome
27. Preventive care and health maintenance
28. Primary and secondary amenorrhea, and hirsutism
29. Psychosomatic problems
30. Recognition and counseling for substance abuse (alcohol, narcotics, etc.)
31. Respiratory tract diseases
32. Sexual assault
33. Sexual dysfunction

34. Sexually transmitted diseases

35. Smoking cessation and treatment of obesity

36. Spousal abuse

37. Ultrasound

38. Urinary Tract Infections

39. Vaginal discharge

40. Vulvar disease

* Recent new categories

It is not necessary, nor have I ever seen anyone use all 40 categories. You get to choose among the 40 categories, so for those unchosen ones, simply list the category on your case list and record "None observed." Remember, you cannot include any patients who appear on the hospital lists. Also include the total number of office ultrasounds that you personally performed in obstetric and gynecologic patients, as well as in other areas (e.g., abdominal, thoracic, pediatric).

*Column confusion* is the <u>most common construction error</u> on the office case list. The *results* column is intended for the results of the treatment, **not** the result of the diagnostic procedure. Think about it. Why would you have to jump two columns over and then back again?

For example, if the problem is a High Grade SIL Pap smear, then your diagnostic procedure is colposcopic directed biopsies, whose results (e.g., ECC negative, ectocervix CIN III) are listed within that diagnostic procedure column. The treatment is then a LEEP, and the pathology (CIS margins clear) is listed in the *results* column.

This concept is better understood if you write it out. Grab a blank office case list sheet and fill in each of the columns. The premise is that we read from left to right and top to bottom. Again, if you list your results for your procedure in the *results* column, the reader has to read through the next column, which is the *treatment* column, to get to the *results* column. He now realizes he needs to disregard and block out the *treatment* column and go back and reread the procedure to match up the results.

Are you confused? You can bet the examiner reading this case list is also. Let's compound the problem. Let's put the results for both the procedures and the treatment in the *results* column. Do you now see the confusion in trying to figure out what results match with what? Hopefully, Examples 4 and 5 on pages 77 and 78 will help you avoid this common mistake.

It's not a "show stopper" if you've made this mistake, since so many others have as well. However, it stands out, in a good sense, when you've done it right, as it gives an impression of attention to detail and methodical and meticulous patient management.

In both the obstetrics and gynecology sections, we discussed that how you word a problem great influences interpretation and your defense. I used the "calling a rose a rose" analogy. I advised using general terms only when you had a large number of cases of the same kind. Since you cannot list more than two patients per category, this does not apply to the office.

Recall the example of menometrorrhagia for the gynecology example. You could have the same problem on the office case list. However, you would not want to list the generic medical therapy as the stand-alone treatment. You would want to be specific, such as progesterone, OCPs, IUD, DMPA, or GnRH agonists.

Don't misinterpret this to mean you cannot use generic concepts. On the contrary, sometimes this can cleverly dodge an unwanted line of questioning. For example, use a generic term for a drug if you want to avoid discussing its specific contents (e.g., hormone replacement therapy rather than Prempro). On the other end of the spectrum, you can use generic terminology to bait questions you do want to discuss, such as antibiotics rather than Cipro.

Unlike the obstetric and gynecologic sections, at least you have a choice in the selection of patients. Use this choice to your strategic advantage for the office practice case list. Carefully organize your office list before you enter the first patient in order to focus your collection of patients. Approach this strategy as you would an investment. How much *risk* are you willing to incur?

If you are a low-risk, conservative type, then choose categories and patients that typify your mode of practice and are textbook examples. The advantage of this approach is that your comfort zone and knowledge base are at their highest and will be the least affected by anxiety under the exam environment. The disadvantage is that you leave the door wide open for the examiners to choose which "oddities" and "aberrations" to your theme they wish to explore.

A speculative, high-risk taker can bait the examiners by listing rare or difficult categories (e.g., sexual dysfunction, pediatric gynecology, primary care topics) or extremes within common categories (e.g., intrauterine insemination for infertility or Müllerian tract abnormality for amenorrhea).

The likelihood that such "oddities" will pique the examiners interest and therefore limit them to your agenda is high. You will be prepared and thus perform well. The disadvantage is that you still need to know the basics; thus, the overall preparation is more involved. Since you are also on the fringe, the examiner may have greater expectations.

Ideally, as with your investment portfolio, your case list should be diversified. In other words, your case list should have a sampling of both types of patients. Keep in mind your strategic objectives as you begin to collect patients. It will be obvious which strategy you should incorporate for most categories and patients.

Because choice is involved, collection of patients in this section is the most prone to procrastination. Keep a list of the 40 categories on your desk and begin to collect representative patients. Since you are limited to two patients per category, stop collecting further patients after you have gathered four names. To avoid an avalanche at the end, begin screening categories for definite "keepers" or "rejects" by six months (November or December). Similarly, three-quarters of the categories should be chosen in the following three months. In the final three months, only the remaining one-quarter needs to be completed.

For the four "keepers" in each category, write a narrative of the patient management issues. Next extract the pertinent data for entry onto the ABOG form. Err on the side of entering too much information initially. It is easier to delete extraneous facts than to search later for incomplete or forgotten details.

## Clinical Summary—Conservative

Patient Joyce Lauden is a 48-year-old 4G/4P who complains of night sweats, mood swings, and irritability. She had a vaginal hysterectomy three years ago for menorrhagia. Her physical exam and past medical history are unremarkable. She has no personal nor family history of gynecologic malignancies. Your diagnosis is perimenopause. You advise her to try an estradiol patch 0.1mg twice weekly. Her symptoms resolve. For the initial ABOG form entry, see Example 6 on page 79.

## Clinical Summary—Speculative

Patient Jennifer Schroeder is a 21-year-old 1G/1P who had an uncomplicated vaginal delivery 18 months ago. She complains of persistent unilateral galactorrhea. She discontinued the OCP six months ago but still has not started her menses. She denies headaches or visual changes. A urine pregnancy test is negative. She has a progestin withdrawal bleed. Thyroid function tests are normal. The prolactin level is moderately elevated (65ng/ml). A prolactin- secreting adenoma is suspected. You recommend an MRI or CT of the sella turcica to determine whether it is a micro- or a macroadenoma. Because she is financially strapped, you settle for an x-ray, which is normal. She is started on Bromocriptine, 1.25 mg q.h.s. x 1 week, then increased to 2.5 mg b.i.d. A repeat prolactin test is normal, and her menses return. For the initial ABOG form entry, see Example 7 on page 79. Your office practice case list should have a variety of styles, ranging from conservative to speculative. The key is to tailor the style which is the most appropriate for each case.

## Peer Review

By this point ,you have become intimately entwined in the nitty-gritty details of each case. You know them almost too well. Not surprisingly, most of us cannot see the forest for the trees. For this reason, it is imperative to enlist the aid of others who can see the big picture. I recommend that you tap into a variety of resources, including specialists, generalists, academicians, non-academicians, peers who know you well, and peers who don't know you at all.

If you are a generalist, it is extremely helpful to seek a specialist's opinion and vice versa. The specialist will more likely reflect the profile of the examiner, yet the generalist will be more familiar with the basic ACOG standards. Regardless, both sides quickly forget the other's unique perspective, especially if practicing in an exclusive environment. You want to critique your case list from as many angles as possible to best anticipate potential questions.

I recommend that you send your obstetrics section to a generalist and/or your referring maternal/fetal medicine specialist; the gynecology section to a generalist, your referring gynecologic oncologist, and/or urogynecologist; and the office practice list to a generalist and/or reproductive endocrinologist and/or family practitioner or internist. In addition, send one or more sections to someone who is familiar with your mode of practice (e.g., your partner or local colleague) as a check for consistency and conformity to your known mode of practice. Finally, send segments to a peer of like profile (e.g., another generalist or same specialist), who is less known to you, to look for glaring mistakes and to evaluate adherence to the ACOG standard of care. A final check can be a professional, such as faculty at a review course, who routinely reviews many case lists.

Remember to give your consultants ample time to review their sections. You must send the sections in sufficient time but make crystal-clear your deadlines. Send the first batch in May or early June and have it due mid-June or no later than July 1. Return revised drafts to them by the second week in July with a due date in the third week of July.

The purpose at this time is to make recommendations for strategic organization of your case list. Return the masterpiece in August or September to help plan its defense. It is ideal but not essential to tap into all of the above resources. It is imperative at least to consult a few. Remember, their job is to give you guidance. You may want to incorporate all, some, or none of their recommendations. Take their advice for what it's worth, but make it worth your while!

## Case List Logistics

Your case list must conform *exactly* to the ABOG specifications. You will receive a package with instructions for preparing the case list after receipt of your application and fee. Keep it readily at hand, for you will refer to it frequently. Do not rely on previous instructions, because instructions change yearly. Check and double-check for compliance each step of the way.

You absolutely—no ifs, ands, or buts—must duplicate the *exact* format of the ABOG forms. You can simply make copies of the original forms and then type in the data. The disadvantage is that this old-fashioned way makes editing difficult and almost always necessitates retyping the whole darn page to make it look acceptable. I recommend instead that you use a computer with a program that *exactly* reproduces the ABOG form. You can either customize your own program (see Appendix D) or use the ABOG case list software.

The case list must be typed with at least 12-point type on 8.5 x 11 inch, unbound white paper. The headings must conform in all details, and you must provide the information indicated by the ABOG format. Every column must be completed.

Your name and case list number must be on every page. You need to identify if you are using senior residency, fellowship, or post residency cases. All case lists must be de-identified, as required by the HIPAA privacy rule, or they will be rejected. If you do not have patients to report in a category at each hospital, still insert the appropriate form in the proper order and specify "None" on the form.

Each section must group overall headings in accordance with the following ABOG dictum:

1. Obstetrical Case List

    I.   Number of Uncomplicated Spontaneous Deliveries—enumerated on page 1

    II.  Obstetrical Categories (1-32)–Starts on page 1

    III. Total number of ultrasound and color Doppler examinations performed by you upon hospitalized obstetrical patients–Enumerated on last page

    IV. Total number of

        A. Apgar scores 5 or less

        B. Infants <2500 grams

        C. Perinatal deaths—Enumerated on last page

2. Gynecological Case List

    I.   Gynecological Categories (1-30)—Starts on page 1

    II.  Total number of ultrasound and color Doppler examinations performed by you upon hospitalized gynecological patients—Enumerated on last page

3. Office Practice Case List

    I.   Office Practice Categories (1-40)—Starts of page 1

    II.  Total number of ultrasound and color Doppler examinations on

        A. Obstetrical patients

        B. Gynecological patients

        C. Other areas such as abdominal, thoracic, pediatric, etc.—Enumerated on last page

Standard nomenclature should be used. *Only* ABOG-approved abbreviations are acceptable (see Appendix A). Practically speaking, it's okay to use well-accepted abbreviations (e.g., HCG for Human Chorionic Gonadotropin). Your non-local reviewer should pick up on local abbreviations that are not universal and therefore should be deleted (e.g., IOL, Induction of Labor). Only the English language is permissible.

The pages of the case list should be numbered consecutively within each section so that each page has a unique number. Likewise, all patients must be numbered consecutively so that each patient also has a unique number.

The hospital number refers to the sequential ordering of hospitals. The summary sheet must contain the combined totals of all hospitals. The affidavit sheet must be signed by the medical records librarian from *each* hospital.

The case list must be arranged in the following order and submitted in triplicate (3 copies):

A.  Summary sheet (7 copies)

B.  Affidavit sheet (for each hospital)

C.  Obstetric patient list for each hospital

D.  Gynecologic patient list for each hospital

E.  Office patient list

If your examination fee has been paid and the three copies of your case list have been received by August 1 and approved by the board, you will receive an admission form and notification of the month your exam. They will not inform you of the date and time until the month prior to your exam.

When you report for your exam, you must bring one *unaltered* copy of your case list. Effective 2008, you may now bring the copy that has the patients' initials. You must also sign a statement on the morning of the exam attesting that you have had no restrictions in your hospital privileges or medical license.

## Strategic Organization of the Case List

The case list is the only exam component that you are allowed to complete ahead of time. As with any take-home test, you are empowered to polish it entirely to your standard. You have the luxury to plan its organization and compose it to your advantage.

Strategy and tactics are defined as the purposeful and deliberate carrying out of intent. Most of us are familiar with these terms as they apply to the military. Strategy is the "why" or intent, and tactics are the "how to" or the steps to carry out the intent.

Strategy and tactics are the root of the basic war dogma, "Know your enemy." To order troops to "take that hill" without regard to strategy and tactics would result in disaster. Battles aren't won simply on paper; they are fought on land, air, and sea. In other words, the battle is carefully studied from all angles to ensure victory before the first soldier bears arms. Your best weapon on this test is your case list. Carefully inspect it from all angles to best plot your strategy. Then employ all necessary tactics to ensure victory.

The first step in analyzing the "enemy" is to understand the reason for the case list. The purpose is to examine your ability to manage patients. You are held to the level of a consultant for non-OB/GYN physicians. Your strategy is to construct a case list that resoundingly reflects your understanding of this expectation.

As long as the case list meets the ABOG requirements, you have considerable freedom to incorporate your strategy. Numerous tactics can be used. The following are by no means all-inclusive; rather, they should serve as catalysts to help you develop your own strategy.

First, take a stance on the detail of your case list. ABOG states that "only pertinent data, not summaries," should be included. Nonetheless, a case list "insufficient in breadth and depth of clinical difficulty" may not be accepted. Furthermore, carelessly prepared or incomplete case lists may contribute to failure on the exam. On the other hand, exhaustive details leave little room for basic management questions and force the examiner to interrogate about trivia.

Thus, the theme for completing the forms is analogous to the advice given to medical students for cutting sutures on their surgical rotations. "Not too long, not too short—just right!" Of course, each staff member has a different preference; therefore, the poor student is always wrong. It isn't long before the student figures out to ask the resident the staff physician's preference before each surgery.

Use the same strategy to tackle your case list. Obtain case lists from previous candidates. Note that there are as many different styles as there are candidates. Furthermore, the depth of information varies with each patient. There is, however, a bell-shaped curve representative of the depth of detail for each case list.

The following examples typify "too long" and "too short" and "just right" detail for most cases. I underscore "most" because clearly there are exceptions. Strategically, you want some cases on the extremes of the bell-shaped curve.

A "just right" case should project a logical sequence of sound patient management consistent with ACOG standards. The detail either satisfies the examiner's need to ask questions or invites a discussion of routine, straightforward topics along any entry of the management algorithm. The theme is "bottom-line up front." Ideally, the majority of your case list is composed of such cases.

In Example 8 (page 79), note that the preoperative diagnosis of an "acute abdomen, but hemodynamically stable" justifies initial use of laparoscopy rather than laparotomy in this surgical emergency. Furthermore, the "suspected cornual pregnancy" was indeed confirmed; thus, the candidate prudently and humbly put down the laparoscope and proceeded with the laparotomy. His surgical decision to resect the cornual ectopic was consistent with the standard of care, and the pathology further supported his preoperative suspicion.

The examiner's questions about the candidate's surgical management of ectopic pregnancy should be answered. If the examiner chooses to ask any questions, they would be generic and related to any step of the algorithm of ectopic pregnancy management. Furthermore, the examiner would probably confine his questions to the basics rather than explore esoteric spin-offs not addressed by the patient (e.g., medical management, risk factors, or recurrence).

A "too long" case can block questions like a "just right" case, but it differs in the degree of detail. A "too long" case has excessive detail, so the few remaining questions are at the end of the spectrum of patient management, dealing with the obscure and little known. A "too long" case list reflects an obsession with minutia that raises doubt as to your ability to see the big picture. Suspicion also arises that the patient is subjected to extraneous and unnecessary lab tests and procedures.

The patient in Example 9 (page 80) is listed under the office category of *Menopausal problems*, yet other non-pertinent issues are raised and hence are fair game for the examiner to address. Enumeration of implied tasks such as "history and physical exam" as well as the conventional screens of "Pap smear, mammogram, and Hemoccult" suggests that the candidate may view them as mandatory for any menopausal patient. Not all of the diagnostic procedures are necessary in every case. No doubt this raises questions of the candidate's ability to recognize basic management issues. Finally, listing brand names of medications mandates justification of the specific brand and hence knowledge of its pharmacology. These unwelcome questions can be avoided entirely by referring instead to the class of drugs (e.g., hormone replacement therapy instead of Premarin and Provera).

On the other hand, "too long" cases can be used to your strategic advantage if they occur sparingly throughout the case list (see Example 10 on page 81). They can block questions on a topic the candidate would rather not discuss. They also can be used as a legal crib sheet for a topic that is not easily remembered. The candidate can flip to the representative patient when the topic arises even if not specifically discussing that patient.

As in the previous example, there are few unanswered questions. The remaining questions are on the fringe and beyond what would be expected for this topic. The candidate clearly followed a logical progression down the workup algorithm. Unlike the previous example, all of the ordered lab tests were necessary. Furthermore, referral to a specialist underscores the candidate's recognition that he or she has reached the extent of his or her abilities and humbly refers the patient's care.

In contrast to a "too long" case, a "too short" case provides insufficient information and obliges the examiner to inquire further. Because minimal information is provided, the examiner can start anywhere on the spectrum of questions. The scarcity of detail also leaves doubts about the thoroughness of the candidate's management. If the bulk of the list exhibits such cases, the examiner is overwhelmed and frustrated as to where to start because there are questions on every case.

In Example 11 (page 82), note that the entire page leaves questions about every patient. The information is so sparse and generic that the examiner could spend the allotted time interrogating the candidate about this page alone. Imagine how the examiner will feel if this page is representative of the entire list! Pity the poor unsuspecting candidate who must face an examiner who is poised for attack.

If, however, "too short" types occur rarely on your case list, the candidate can bait the examiner to open discussion of a topic that the candidate wants to discuss. Because the information is sparse, the examiner most likely will start at the beginning and say, "Tell me about this patient." At this point, the candidate is in the driver's seat.

As in the previous example, Example 12 (page 83) leaves many questions unanswered. Note, however, that this topic is unusual, far from the mainstream "bread-and-butter" topics. It is strategically worded so that the only logical question is to start at the beginning: "What happened?" or "Tell me about this patient." The candidate's control of the opening question drives subsequent ones that the candidate anticipated and is well prepared to answer. Note also that the candidate can buy a lot of time while scoring big.

On the same theme of volume is the concept of redundancy on the office practice case list. Remember, this is the only one of the three sections that you can choose the patients. Recall also that you can list no more than two for each category.

I often will see candidates list essentially the same case, but two different patients for one category. For example, in the vaginal discharge category, you list two patients, each with yeast vaginitis—same problem, same procedure, same treatment, and of course the same result as both got better. I am stumped with this strategy. Is it because you really want to talk about this topic? How exciting are two yeast infections? I think it is a waste of a patient and category and gives a cookie cutter impression.

If you're going to chose two patients for the same category, I recommend they be two different themes within that category. Back to our vaginal discharge example, at least make one patient with acute candidiasis and the other chronic. Better yet, choose two different discharges completely, say one with yeast and the other with trichomonas or bacterial vaginosis.

In addition to the volume of data, there is considerable strategy in the wording of cases. Tailor each case to your objective. For example, on the obstetrics case list, you may elect to simply list "routine hemorrhage management" in the *treatment* column for the complication of postpartum bleeding. This wording is generic and therefore begs a general question, whereas if the treatment was more extreme (such as culminating in a hysterectomy) you may want to be specific to justify why you elected that modality of therapy.

Another similar debate is with the wording for fetal distress. I'm sure you know that listing "fetal distress" as an antepartum complication is a no-no. Typically, you should replace "fetal distress" with "non-reassuring fetal heart rate tracing" or "fetal intolerance to labor." Exceptions would include clarifying a modality of treatment. For example, use "repetitive variable decelerations" if you performed an amnioinfusion, or "terminal bradycardia" for an emergent operative delivery, or "fetal tachycardia" for chorioamnionitis. Likewise, your treatment for any of the above could generically be listed simply as "intrauterine fetal resuscitation," although sometimes you may want to specify if you performed a scalp or cord pH, fetal scalp electrode, fetal scalp stimulation or an amnioinfusion.

After you're satisfied with the volume, categories, and wording for each case, consider the order in which to list the patients. Chronologic order is straightforward but does not take advantage of strategic posturing within each section. The ABOG program lumps patients by procedures. The disadvantage is that the examiner can search out the worst or most complicated patient within each procedure type in just seconds. As of 2000, patients have to be categorized by procedure. Although this requirement strips away some latitude, there is still room for creative strategic placement of cases.

Put your best foot, or at least case, forward. In other words, list your best cases first under their respective category. What the heck. Why not strategically use **bold**, CAPITALIZE, or *italicize* key words to catch the examiner's eye, so he doesn't miss them?

Note carefully that a *best* case is not necessarily synonymous with flawless management and perfect outcome. *Best* implies a case that you know cold and are the best prepared to defend. A best case may be a case from hell, but it demonstrates your flexibility, quick thinking, humbleness in calling for help, or acknowledging error and henceforth changing a mode of practice.

An experienced and clever examiner will not be fooled by any order of listing of patients. Regardless of their location, know your worst cases best. Obviously, spread them out, with an ideal limit of one per page. Try not to put similar complications close together to avoid their jumping out on a skim-through. The exception is a recurrent complication that finally motivated you to change your mode of practice. Make it clear that you tracked the outcomes, recognized the redundancy of your error, and fixed it with resulting good outcomes.

All case lists should have some poor outcomes or complications. No one is perfect. As a matter of fact, a case list lacking an occasional complication is highly suspicious for willful withholding and may prompt ABOG to verify its authenticity.

Fraudulent case lists result in suspension from the exam. That's bad, but remember that the worse part is that it will follow you the rest of your career. Every single time you renew your medical licenses or hospital privileges, you are asked, "Has there ever been any disciplinary action taken against you?" Remember, you also had your medical records director sign a notarized copy verifying the authenticity of your case list. This will also reflect poorly on your admitting hospital. Bottom line, don't even think about withholding any cases. You will woefully regret it your entire career.

In conclusion, the time spent to plan the organization of your case list is enormous. Certainly, it is logistically easier to list the patients chronologically or to let the computer program dictate their order. But the potential gain in strategically ordering the cases is far greater than the time invested, as repeatedly confirmed by previous candidates reflecting on what they would do differently. A resounding response is "organize my case list better," for they know, as will you come August 1, that your case list is cast in stone.

## Editing

Although the time frame for when the case list is due (August 1) relative to when its compilation is completed (June 30) is tight, there is time for at least one revision and perhaps more. One of the biggest regrets of previous candidates is running out of time to better organize and edit their case list. A carefully composed case list is by far easier to defend than a case list haphazardly thrown together. Besides, a mere six weeks of intense effort is minute compared with the year invested in its compilation.

Implementing your strategy during the compilation of the case list maximizes the efficiency of editing. However, the gestalt of the case list is not obvious until the first typewritten draft. Critique the case list from the examiner's viewpoint. Look at it first from a distance, then up close. Your peers should afford you the same favor. The easiest facet of editing the big picture is the physical layout. Make sure it is reader-friendly. Esthetics that appease the reader's eye include the following:

1. Use a conventional, easy-to-read font in sharp, dark, black ink.

2. The letters should be large enough to avoid eye strain (at least 12-point type). Remember, most of your examiners wear bifocals. An average page has four to six patients (see Examples 13 and 14 on pages 84 and 85).

3. The layout should enable readers to delineate between cases and assist them in following the flow of management within each case. This is facilitated by:
   - Highlighting or shadowing category headings
   - Leaving space between patients
   - Placing vertical tracking lines to demarcate columns
   - Placing horizontal tracking lines to follow flow within and between columns

Verify that the mandatory objective data are included:

1. Within each section, the columns should contain the required information:

   a. Summary Sheet: verifying that the numbers are correct

   b. De-identified hospital and patient #

   c. Obstetrics
      - Unique case list # and page #
      - Gravida and parity only

- EGA in whole numbers
- Friedman terminology for dysfunctional labor, not FTP (optional) (see Example 15 on page 86)

d. Gynecology

- Size (cm) of ovarian cysts
- Surgical pathology weight of uterus (gm)
- Cytology for Pap smears in SIL terminology and histology for biopsies in CIN (optional)
- Endometrial hyperplasia with or without atypia (optional)
- Leiomyomata, not fibroids (optional)
- Abnormal uterine bleeding or specifics (e.g., menometrorrhagia), not dysfunctional uterine bleeding

e. Office practice

- 40 patients total
- Maximum of two patients per category
- Do not duplicate patients that also appear on the OB or GYN lists.

2. Laboratory values with appropriate units

3. Use ABOG-approved abbreviations only (see Appendix A)

4. Absolutely no typographical errors

5. Minimize grammatical errors

Now step back and look for trends. To do so, answer the following questions:

1. Have you put your best foot forward? In other words, are your *best* cases listed first in each category?

2. Have you limited significant complications and worst cases to one per page?

3. Have you spread out like complications and avoided listing them consecutively?

4. Does each page have a variety of patient management themes?

5. Does each page vary in complexity?

6. Is the case list mode of practice consistent with how you actually practice?

Finally, get out the microscope and analyze each case for the following:

1. Can the examiner clearly follow your flow of patient management? (see Examples 16 and 17 on pages 87 and 88). This is of paramount importance on the obstetrics and office list, where column confusion makes all the difference. Refer again to Example 1 on page 75 and Examples 4 and 5 on pages 77 and 78. Additionally, each topic on the obstetrics case list should be organized chronologically, and the management of each topic should flow left to right. In other words, the reader should see Problem A in the *antepartum* column and see the matching treatment directly to the right in the *operative procedures* and/or *treatment* column. If Problem A occurred first in the pregnancy, then it should be listed before problems that developed later.

2. Are the majority of cases "just right" in volume (pertinent data, not summaries)? (See Example 18 on page 89.)

3. Are there only a few "too long" and "too short" cases? Do they meet your strategic objective?

4. Do all cases meet the ACOG standard of care? If not, justify why.

5. How does the wording generate topics? Is it consistent with your intended strategy?

If you have followed each of the above steps, then your case list is ready to be submitted. Although theoretically each draft can be edited, the impact declines exponentially with the number of revisions beyond two. Furthermore, the clock is ticking, and time will be up. Push for at least one rewrite. Two edits are ideal but difficult, given the time constraints. Nonetheless, a comparison of your original draft with your masterpiece makes all of the time and effort well worth the blood, sweat, and tears. After all, better now than after the test.

## Using the Case List as a Study Tool

You must know your case list *cold* to pass the exam. This dogma is steadfastly affirmed by successful candidates, regardless of when they took the exam. One way to meet this mandate and tackle your list of study topics (see Chapter 8) as well is to organize your studies around your case list. There will be some overlap of topics; therefore, this system is not as time-intensive as it initially seems.

First, obtain three large three-ring binders for each of the three sections. Then, for every patient draft a narrative summary of the management issues as if you were presenting her at morning report or teaching rounds. Examples for each of the three sections of the case list were cited earlier (see pages 40-51). Next, file her prenatal record, delivery note, and discharge summary.

Now identify the issues that are raised by this case, and couple each topic with the pertinent reference(s) from the *ACOG Compendium*. Try to limit your review to this resource. Rarely does the *Compendium* not have a reference on a topic. In this case, next check the *ACOG Precis* and, as a last resort, other references. Be disciplined, and extract only relevant issues. File these behind the hospital records.

Finally, put yourself in the examiner's shoes and brainstorm what questions may be asked. Consider questions directly related to each patient as well as spin-off topics. Verify your hunches by cross-referencing topics raised by your peers and especially in mock oral exams.

Here is an example of how to use your case list as a study tool:

**Case list—Patient No. 124** (Example 18 on page 89)

**Clinical summary:** L.V. is a 30-year-old 2G/1P whose pregnancy was complicated by maternal obesity and a 40-lb weight gain. An ultrasound obtained at 38 weeks estimated fetal weight of 4000 grams. Her first stage of labor was 8 hours, and her second stage was 45 minutes.

**Primary clinical issue:** Shoulder dystocia

**Spin-off topics:** Macrosomia, maternal obesity, weight gain in pregnancy, gestational diabetes, ultrasonography, dysfunctional labor, induction/augmentation of labor, FHR monitoring, obstetrical anesthesia, operative vaginal deliveries, and episiotomy.

**ACOG Compendium references:** *Shoulder Dystocia*—Practice Bulletin #40, 2002; *Operative Vaginal Delivery*—Practice Bulletin #17, 2000; *Fetal Macrosomia*—Practice Bulletin #22, 2000; *Induction of Labor*—Practice Bulletin #10, 1999; *Gestational Diabetes*—Practice Bulletin #30, 2001; *Obstetric Analgesia and Anesthesia*—Practice Bulletin #36, 2002; *Dystocia and the Augmentation of Labor*—Practice Bulletin #40, 2003; *Ultrasonography in Pregnancy*—Practice Bulletin #58, 2004; *Intrapartum Fetal Heart Rate Monitoring*—Practice Bulletin #70, 2005; *Episiotomy*—Practice Bulletin #71, 2006.

You have accomplished many goals by this tactic. No doubt you now know the patient cold! You have also reviewed at least ten topics that surely were on your study list. Finally, your brainstorming of potential questions has better enabled you to defend your management and discuss related topics.

## Defending Your Case List

Forewarned is forearmed. In other words, preparedness is your best defense. For this exam, ideal preparedness implies that the examiner actually asks the questions that you predicted.

The secret is to determine which questions the examiner will ask. Remember that the purpose of the case list is to examine your ability to manage patients. This requires validating your knowledge of the basic clinical sciences, but especially your ability to apply that knowledge to the practice of medicine. You know your case list better than anyone. Hence you are probably the toughest critic of all. **If you were the examiner, what questions would you ask?**

To prepare your defense, step into the examiner's shoes. Pick up someone else's case list and look at it. Note that after just a few minutes you already have an image of its owner. The components of the first impression based on your case list are no different from the components in meeting someone.

Surprisingly, the bulk of the first impression is based on appearance. In other words, "It's not what you say, but how you say it." The case list's first impression is based on its physical layout and organization. Of course, you can't judge a book by its cover. Therefore, the examiners will then peruse the list for generalities to get a feel for the candidate's mode of practice and whether it conforms to the ACOG standard of care. Finally, the examiners will select individual cases for questioning to validate their hunches.

Now tackle your case list with these three components in mind: first impression, general themes/trends, and specific cases that stand out. A formula for this process is described in the previous discussion concerning editing. Obviously, the best defense is to organize the list strategically so that it best withstands the brunt of the examiner's offense. Once the case list is submitted, however, it is set in stone. Now you must defend "the writing on the wall." This is how:

Start by determining your case list's first impression. The Summary Sheet is the most telling for the obstetrics and gynecology sections, for a number of reasons. The volume of patients within each category is the most revealing element. The numbers indicate experience, complication rate, mode of practice, and adherence to the ACOG standard of care.

In the obstetrics section, the total number of deliveries, which is the summation of total cases and total uncomplicated spontaneous deliveries, reveals how busy you are. The average number of deliveries is 75-150. Significant deviation, such as <50 or > 200, raises concern that you are either not busy enough or too busy to optimally maintain your technical skills and clinical judgment. You must have a ready explanation to justify the extremes (e.g., > 200—MFM specialist, joined a busy practice; < 50—started a rural solo practice, extended maternity leave).

Next, calculate your primary and repeat cesarean section rate. The summary sheet no longer has a category just for this, so it takes a motivated examiner to extract out the numbers. Make it easy and be ready for him. You also must be able to defend your math (the components of the denominator). The average rate on most case lists is 20-35%. Significant deviation such as < 10% or > 50% suggests poor judgment in criteria selection for cesarean delivery. Justify exceptional rates (e.g., > 30% MFM at a tertiary center with preterm deliveries or no VBACs in a rural setting secondary to lack of anesthesia availability or maternal requests for elective CDs; <10% low-risk obstetrics practice in a rural setting).

The remaining rates that can be calculated have less defined values. Examples include VBAC and induction rates. As noted above, extremes are a red flag. Traditionally, too few VBACs were a red flag. Given the increasing complications of vaginal deliveries after a prior cesarean delivery, the pendulum is swinging back in favor of elective repeat cesarean deliveries. A low VBAC rate may be a marker that the patient is counseled with prejudice to dissuade her from trying labor. On the other end of the spectrum, a high elective induction rate, particularly at gestational ages < 39 weeks, raises suspicions that convenience rather than sound medical judgment drive your decision making. Similarly, the number of vacuum or forceps deliveries is not eye-catching unless it is excessive. A random check verifies that they are used appropriately (e.g., rare mid-pelvic deliveries or rotations).

Few or absent breech deliveries cue questions about the steps of a breech delivery. On the other hand, the national trend is to deliver breeches by cesarean section, in spite of ACOG's recent endorsement for vaginal breech deliveries. Thus, fewer than two vaginal breech deliveries trigger the examiner to scrutinize your competency to practice this fading art. Obviously, the safest route for both the mom and baby is a vertex vaginal delivery. Thus, expect questions on external cephalic versions: counseling, candidates, contraindications, technique and success rates. A nice way to block this question is simply to make an annotation such as "failed/refused-declined/successful ECV" in the *antepartum complications* column.

A high number of obstetric ultrasounds may prompt questions about your technical proficiency and quality control measures. A quick glance at the *Apgars below 5*, *perinatal deaths*, and *postpartum admission* columns prompts a quick search in the case list for the corresponding case.

Attention to detail and precise terminology blocks out questions, scores points for style, and satisfies the examiner's concern for a level of understanding on a topic. Under the abnormal fetal growth category, preface IUGR with symmetric or asymmetric. All too often, we get sloppy with the breakdown of hypertensive disorders by using the antiquated term of pregnancy induced rather than gestational hypertension or qualifying preeclampsia with nonexistent nomenclature of mild or moderate.

It's best to call a spade a spade. In other words, if your induction was truly elective, then word it accordingly in the *antepartum complications* column. Refer to *Induction of Labor*—ACOG Practice Bulletin #10, 1999 for ACOG-appropriate indications for induction. Impending/suspected macrosomia as an indication for induction, although commonplace, lacks evidence, and will only get you into a miserable discussion of scientific interpretation of the literature as well as trying to justify a breach of ACOG standard of care.

You know the expected questions for certain topics, so just cut to the chase. In multifetal pregnancy, make sure to specify twins or other, the chorion and amnion status, and presentation at deliver (e.g., vertex/vertex). On operative vaginal deliveries, absolutely specify outlet or low.

In perusing the gynecology section, the examiner will again first check the numbers. Reportedly, you must do at least eight of a particular procedure annually to maintain your skills. Historically, vaginal hysterectomies fall into this category for many candidates. This prompts the order, "Dictate the steps of a VH."

Similarly, the examiner will search the indications for your abdominal hysterectomies to make sure that they could not have been attempted vaginally in the first place. Some common reasons to support why the patient was not a VH candidate include nulliparity, inadequate uterine descensus, contracted pelvis, prior multiple cesarean sections, enlarged uterus, history of PID, or suspected endometriosis. Thus, make your wording clear in the *preoperative diagnosis* column to defend your indication for your route of hysterectomy. Check the parity and weights first to make sure you don't look silly. Specifically, to use the excuse of lack of descensus in a multiparous patient or to state the uterus was enlarged for a uterus less than 200 grams will backfire on you.

On the same theme, you must be able to defend the indications for your laparoscopic assisted hysterectomies. First, use the appropriate definitions for laparoscopic assisted vaginal hysterectomy (LAVH), laparoscopic supracervical hysterectomy (LSH), and a total laparoscopic hysterectomy (LSH). Hopefully, your case list doesn't have all laparoscopic hysterectomies or you will look like a "one surgery for all" surgeon.

The alarming complication rate and the national decline in residency training of vaginal surgery has sparked a national debate. The concern is that the LAVH is inappropriately substituted to compensate for inadequate vaginal surgical skills. The above list that excludes a patient as a VH candidate applies only partially to the LAVH patient. Lack of descensus or an inadequate pelvic outlet cannot be overcome by the laparoscope unless you perform a LSH or TLH. A uterine specimen weight less than 200 grams does not support your contention that an enlarged uterus prohibited attempting a VH. It also raises doubt of your pelvic exam abilities.

Furthermore, desire for a BSO should not be the only indication for an LAVH. A competent vaginal surgeon should be able to remove the ovaries at least 60-70% of the time. Only if you are unsuccessful should you complete the procedure laparoscopically. To subject the majority of patients to what applies only to the minority makes no sense and suggests that the surgeon lacks confidence.

Finally, an excessive number of operative laparoscopies is suggestive of a "cowboy." You must demonstrate clinical judgment in your selection criteria of the appropriate route of surgery. Unless you have a predominance of vaginal hysterectomies, you can expect a question on your thought process for choosing the route of hysterectomy and how you counsel the patient on the risks/benefits/alternatives for each route. You're golden if your case list has a blend of all the types of hysterectomies.

The Council on Resident Education in Obstetrics and Gynecology (CREOG) mandated the inclusion of urogynecology in the OB/GYN residency training in the mid-1990s. Although I still see many case lists that include *no* urogynecologic procedures, feedback from candidates since the mid-1990s confirms that essentially all of them were asked some questions about urogynecology. As a matter of fact, ABOG has expanded to four categories where urogynecologic questions can pop up: defects in pelvic floor, rectovaginal or urinary tract fistula, urinary and fecal incontinence (operative management), and urinary incontinence (medical management). Just the fact that these categories exist is justification alone to prompt a line of questions, so don't think you're off the hook if you don't have any patients in these categories.

A reasonable line of questioning is how do you support your vaginal cuff in a routine vaginal hysterectomy to prevent prolapse in the first place? Of course, you can allay the examiner's concern by simply listing this in your treatment column, so rather than listing only a vaginal hysterectomy, you may also add Mayo/McCall cul-de-plasty or uterosacral ligament shortening/suspension.

But the question doesn't end there. How does your approach change if the indication is procidentia? Traditionally, the examiner will give you his pen and ask you to draw your initial incision. The answer is "anteriorly at the supravaginal septum at the cervicovaginal junction, since the ureters are saggy posteriorly in the setting of prolapse."

Of course, then, how are you going to support the apex in the setting of prolapse? Make sure you refer to *Pelvic Organ Prolapse* in ACOG Practice Bulletin #85, 2007. The technique you use for a routine, non-prolapsed hysterectomy is not sufficient. Your options are uterosacral shortening and suspension, sacrospinous ligament fixation, abdominal colposacropexy, or a total vaginal mesh/graft. Brace yourself: Historically, this prompts questions on the technique of a sacrospinous ligament fixation. You can reply that hardly anyone, especially your urogynecologist, performs this antiquated technique, but that doesn't get you off the hook. Until this changes, suck it in and be able to describe the technique in great detail, including intraoperative and postoperative complications.

Along the lines of prolapse, you must be prepared for questions on incontinence, both urinary and fecal. You first need to describe the preoperative work up. *Urinary Incontinence* in ACOG Practice Bulletin #63, 2005, does not support fancy multichannel urodynamic testing in the uncomplicated patient, so be prepared to discuss what anyone can perform right there in the office.

The exam focus is on how to treat and prevent urinary incontinence. You must be able to counsel the patient on her options. Absolutely you have to be able to describe in detail at least one of those procedures, including intraoperative and postoperative complications. If you truly don't perform these surgeries, call your local generalist or urogynecologist and observe these procedures. If you can see it in your mind's eye, it will be much easier to defend and especially to think on your feet during the exam.

Another red flag is too many induced abortions. This finding is particularly worrisome for pregnancies greater than 12 weeks, especially if they are elective. As you can imagine, this is a delicate political topic. They will not question the ethics, but will focus on your technique.

Many are no longer performing any oncology cases. It's kind of difficult to defend, with all the evidence showing that patient mortality is lower in the specialist's hands. Thus, I am seeing more case lists with a big fat zero in the invasive carcinoma category for those practitioners in community hospitals who do not have an oncologist on hand. As a matter of fact, there are rare questions on staging, so, as you may have guessed, this does not get you off the hook if you have no patients in this category. The goal now is making sure you don't get caught with your pants down. In other words, how do you carefully work up a patient to ensure that you don't get to the OR and have the pathology come back with an unexpected malignancy?

In addition to the total number of procedures, other categories on the Summary Sheet are revealing. Examiners will search out hospital stays longer than seven days. All they have to do is thumb down the *Days in Hospital* column. They can find the longer stays in a heartbeat, regardless of where they are hidden. Be prepared to defend why your patient required a lengthy hospital stay.

Other categories to be prepared for, even if you don't have any, are those with complications: post-op fever, thromboembolism, and wound healing. You need to be able to recognize, work up, and manage these complications. In 2008, preoperative evaluation of coexisting conditions (respiratory, cardiac, and metabolic diseases) made its debut. This again reflects that swing of the pendulum back to what a gynecologist needs to know about medical issues so as not to get caught unawares.

Note that all three sections require you to list the number of office and inpatient ultrasounds that you personally performed. This new statistic appeared in 2000. Feedback suggests that a high number is a red flag.

If you perform obstetric ultrasounds, make sure that you refer to *Ultrasonography in Pregnancy* in ACOG Practice Bulletin #58, 2004, and to *Performance and Interpretation of Imaging Studies by the Obstetrician/ Gynecologist* in Committee Opinion #243, 2000. You will be asked point blank if you perform or recommend routine screening ultrasounds. They are still not endorsed by ACOG, which recommends ultrasound only if indicated. (This remains controversial.) You should be able to cite a long list of such medical indications.

You should also be aware of the levels of obstetric ultrasounds and their components. Contrary to popular usage, there is no official terminology of a level I, II, or III ultrasound. Rather, the three levels are basic, comprehensive, and limited. The components of a basic ultrasound include the following:

• Fetal number
• Fetal presentation
• Documentation of fetal lie
• Placental location
• Assessment of amniotic fluid volume
• Assessment of gestational age
• Survey of fetal anatomy for *gross* malformations
• Evaluation for maternal pelvic masses

A detailed or targeted ultrasound is performed and interpreted by specially-trained personnel proficient in the detection and recognition of a physiologically or anatomically defective fetus. If you profess to be such an expert, expect technical questions about the specific components within the anatomic survey. On the other hand, know when it is judicious to offer a limited ultrasound only. Common reasons include the following:

• Assessment of amniotic fluid volume
• Fetal biophysical profile testing
• Ultrasonography-guided amniocentesis
• External cephalic version
• Confirmation of fetal viability
• Localization of the placenta in antepartum hemorrhage
• Confirmation of fetal presentation

Similarly, if you perform gynecologic ultrasounds, be familiar with ACOG Technical Bulletin 215, *Gynecologic Ultrasonography* 1995. The most common test topic is determining when to do a transvaginal vs. a transabdominal ultrasound. Secondly, be prepared to expound on which ultrasound features of an adnexal mass are characteristic of benign vs. malignant lesions. Bear in mind that ACOG does not support routine ultrasound screening for ovarian cancer. Finally, expect some technical questions about how to diagnose an ectopic pregnancy.

You must be prepared for questions about ultrasound technique and interpretation if you include ultrasounds in your summary sheet. It is highly likely that you will get some of the above questions if you performed both obstetric and gynecologic ultrasounds. Definitely be prepared to also discuss your quality control measures. On the other hand, if you don't have any ultrasounds reported, you can expect basic or generic questions, if any.

The Summary Sheet gives examiners the most bang for their buck because the facts are right in the open. Next they will hone in closer. They will skim through the case list to get a gestalt of the clinical style.

The physical layout and organization of the case list give the initial impression of your attention to detail. Examiners will conduct a quick check to see whether it is reader-friendly, organized, and free of spelling and grammatical errors and whether it conforms to the ABOG requirements. The examiner's checklist is similar to the one described in the discussion of editing. Remember that the examiner receives your case list before he meets you, so don't underscore the impact this makes and how it can influence the examiner's questions.

The gynecologic section is the easiest to evaluate for attention to detail. Examiners will search out your youngest patient undergoing a hysterectomy. You will need to justify her hysterectomy, especially if her gravida and parity are low. The postoperative pathology should agree with your preoperative diagnosis. For example, if you performed a hysterectomy for abnormal uterine bleeding secondary to uterine leiomyomata and the postoperative pathology showed a normal uterus, you need to explain why.

Likewise, hysterectomies for the mere presence of leiomyomata are not indicated. Justify the hysterectomy with complications from leiomyomata, such as menorrhagia unresponsive to hormonal therapy or D&C.

If you perform incidental appendectomies, you need to justify why. Expect questions about the anatomy and blood supply of the appendix and postoperative complications. On the same theme, an incidental hysterectomy during concurrent prolapse surgery is controversial. You can avoid this topic if you have an appropriate indication for the hysterectomy or if the patient at least also has symptomatic uterine prolapse. Finally, if you performed a procedure for chronic pelvic pain or an adnexal mass, be prepared to list the differential diagnosis.

After examiners have a feel for the case list, they will zero in on individual cases. The obvious red flag is a case with complications. Each examiner has his or her own agenda and style. Remember to think first of horses rather than zebras when you hear hoof beats. In other words, the examiner will most likely start at the top rather than the bottom of the patient management algorithm. Plan your defense accordingly. Approach each case as described earlier in the discussion of using your case list as a study tool (page 63). Identify the main patient management issue or "bottom-line up front." Prepare first for the obvious, then work your way down the flow chart. Save preparation for the esoteric for last, if at all.

Finally, I want to end this chapter where we started. I want to drive home the fact that your best defense is predicting your exam questions. Remember, defending your case list is only a half hour for each section. Although 30 minutes will seem like an eternity, it does limit the number of cases that can be covered. Feedback from both candidates and past examiners confirm the examiners most definitely have an agenda and a set order of questions.

With that in mind, I recommend you pick out the ten cases that you would ask about if you were the examiner. Better yet, ask at least three other colleagues the same question. We all have our own reasons for selecting those ten. Those reasons include complications, a topic of personal interest, a challenging diagnostic dilemma, a technically difficult case, or an unusual or esoteric subject, to name a few. Regardless of the rationale, you will see that at least five cases overlap on everyone's list. You can bet those are going to be on your examiner's list too.

So obviously the more opinions and lists you gather, the better you will be able to fine tune those top ten cases. Once you narrow those down, really dissect them from every angle. Again, enlist your colleagues' help and come up with as many questions as possible. Surely, you will then have thought of most, or at least the magical 70%, of the same questions as the examiner.

Remember to confine your preparation to a review. The ACOG *Compendium* is the best resource to keep you on track. You are expected to demonstrate a level of knowledge similar to other board-certified obstetricians and gynecologists. Once you have reached this level, the examiner will move quickly to the next question.

No doubt, examiners will sometimes drive you beyond the pass threshold. They may want to explore your depth of understanding of a particular topic. More likely, they simply want to verify that you will acknowledge your limitations.

A final preparation tool is a systematic review of your case list. Highlight common ground topics for all cases with a different color. Common ground topics would include the pathophysiology, etiology, or definition for a disease, work-up (labs and radiology), and medications. For example, let's say you use green to highlight any medication on your list. This is your cue to then know the active ingredient or content for a brand name or generic drug, its mechanism of action, indications/contraindications, dosing, side effects, and antidote.

In conclusion, your best defense is to be prepared. Your first line of defense is a strategically constructed case list. Your main defense, then, is to be prepared for the questions you have anticipated. The secret is your accuracy in predicting these questions. The more your case list is critiqued and the more mock oral exams you take, the better your chances of uncovering likely questions. Thus, when it is finally exam time, you will be answering questions that you have already heard many times before.

Example 1    Confusion Complications Column

| # | Pt # No. | Age | Gravida | Para | Gest. Age | Complications | | | Days in Hosp. | Newborn | | | | Days in Hosp. |
| | | | | | | Antepartum | Delivery or Postpartum | Operative Procedures and/ or Treatment | | Complications | Wgt. | Apgar 1 & 5 Minutes | |
|---|---|---|---|---|---|---|---|---|---|---|---|---|---|
| 16 | A16 284486024 | 27 | 4 | 3 | 38 | AI GDM | Protracted labor Nonreassuring FHR | Routine diabetic care. Pitocin augmentation CD | 3 | None | 3760 | 9/9 | 5 |

Example 2    Clinical Summary Extract and First Draft of ABOG Form

| # | Pt & Hospital No. | Age | Gravida | Para | Gest. Age | Complications | | | Days in Hosp. | Newborn | | | | Days in Hosp. |
| | | | | | | Antepartum | Delivery or Postpartum | Operative Procedures and/ or Treatment | | Complications | Wgt. | Apgar 1 & 5 Minutes | |
|---|---|---|---|---|---|---|---|---|---|---|---|---|---|
| 42 | Karen Burke 652688 | 34 | 2 | 0 | 38 | Chronic hypertension Superimposed severe preeclampsia Arrest of dilation | None | Anti-hypertensives Magnesium Sulfate Prostaglandin cervical ripening Pitocin induction Intrauterine press catheter Primary CD | 4 | None | 3435 | 9 & 10 | 3 |

Example 3   Clinical Summary Extract and Initial Entry

| # | Initials & Hosp. No. | Age | Gravida | Para | Diagnostics Preoperative or Admission (Include size of ovarian cysts | Treatment | Surgical Pathology Diagnosis (uterine weight in grams | Complications (Include blood transfusions) | Days in Hosp. |
|---|---|---|---|---|---|---|---|---|---|
| 52 | Joyce Collins | 42 | 2 | 3 | Menorrhagia unresponsive to hormonal therapy | Hysteroscopic-guided fractional dilatation and currettage | Secretory endometrium Endocervix-benign | None | 0 |
| | | | | | Leiomyomata with menorrhagia unresponsive to hormones and dilatation and currettage | Vaginal hysterectomy | Uterus-200 grams leiomyomata cervix-benign | None | 3 |

Example 4   Office Column Confusion  WRONG WAY

## List of Office Practice Patients

*Post Residency Cases
July 1, 200_ – June 30, 200_
Page 1

Candidate's Name:
Caselist Number:

| # | Age | Grav | Para | Problem | Diagnostic Procedures | Treatment | Results | Number of visits |
|---|-----|------|------|---------|----------------------|-----------|---------|------------------|
| 1 | 28 | 2 | 2 | HGSIL Pap smear | Colposcopy | LEEP | ECC – negative<br>Ectocervix – CIN III<br>CIS – margins clear | |

77

Example 5   Office Column Confusion   RIGHT WAY

## List of Office Practice Patients

Candidate's Name:

Caselist Number:

*Post Residency Cases

July 1, 200_ — June 30, 200_

Page 1

| # | A g e | G r a v | P a r a | Problem | Diagnostic Procedures | Treatment | Results | Number of visits |
|---|---|---|---|---|---|---|---|---|
| 1 | 28 | 2 | 2 | HG SIL Pap smear | Colposcopy<br>ECC – negative<br>Ectocervix – CIN III | LEEP | CIS – margins clear | 2 |

78

### Example 6  Clinical Summary—Conservative

| # | Initials & Hosp. No. | Age | Gravida | Para | Problem | Diagnostic Procedures | Treatment | Results | No. of Visits |
|---|---|---|---|---|---|---|---|---|---|
| | Joyce Lauden | 48 | 4 | 4 | Vasomotor symptoms Mood lability | None | Hormone replacement therapy | Resolution of symptoms | 3 |

### Example 7  Office Practice Clinical Summary Speculative

| # | Initials | Age | Gravida | Para | Problem | Diagnostic Procedures | Treatment | Results | No. of Visits |
|---|---|---|---|---|---|---|---|---|---|
| | J.S. | 21 | 1 | 1 | Secondary amenorrhea, galactorrhea | Urinary pregnancy test (normal) Progesterone challenge (withdrawal bleed) Thyroid-stimulating hormone (normal) Prolactin level (elevated) Coned x-ray sella turcica (normal) | Oral contraceptive pills Bromocriptine | Prolactin-secreting pituitary micro-adenoma Return of menses Repeat prolactin (normal) | 3 |

### Example 8  "Just Right"

| # | Initials & Hosp. No. | Age | Gravida | Para | Diagnosis Preoperative or Admission | Treatment | Surgical Pathology Diagnosis | Complications | Days in Hospital |
|---|---|---|---|---|---|---|---|---|---|
| | CM 496264 | 27 | 5 | 2 | Acute abdomen, hemodynamically stable Ectopic pregnancy, (suspected comual) | Laparoscopy Laparotomy Wedge resection of left comua | Comual ectopic pregnancy | None | 1 |

Example 9  "Too Long" – The Wrong Way

| # | Initials | Age | Gravida | Para | Problem | Diagnostic Procedures | Treatment | Results | No. of Visits |
|---|----------|-----|---------|------|---------|----------------------|-----------|---------|---------------|
| | J.L. | 48 | 4 | 4 | Night sweats<br>Mood lability<br>Hypermenorrhea<br>Smoker<br>Obese<br>Decreased libido | History and physical exam<br>Pap smear<br>Mammogram<br>Hemoccult screening<br>Bone densitometry<br>Endometrial biopsy (Dyssynchronous endometrium)<br>Estradiol<br>FSH, LH | Smoking cessation counseling<br>Weight loss counseling<br>Referral to sexual therapist<br>Premarin 1.25 mg P.O. q D<br>Provera 5 mg P.O. q D x 12 q mo | Decrease in smoking<br>5 lb weight loss<br>Resolution of peri-menopausal symptoms | 3 |

Example 10 "Too Long" — The Right Way

| # | Initials | Age | Gravida | Para | Problem | Diagnostic Procedures | Treatment | Results | No. of Visits |
|---|----------|-----|---------|------|---------|----------------------|-----------|---------|---------------|
| 6 | C.E. | 26 | 5 | 1 | Habitual aborter (first trimester) | Products of conception, karyotype (normal) Cervical cultures (normal) Hysterosalpingogram (normal) Immunologic evaluation initial screen: ANA (normal) APTT (normal) Anti-cardiolipin (minimally elevated) Lymphocytotoxic antibodies ordered Thyroid function tests (normal) | Referral to reproductive endocrinologist | Referral pending | 4 |

## Example 11 "Too Short" — The Wrong Way

| # | Initials & Hosp. No. | Age | Gravida | Para | Gest. Age | Complications | | Operative Procedures and/ or Treatment | Days in Hosp. | Newborn | | | | Days in Hosp. |
|---|---|---|---|---|---|---|---|---|---|---|---|---|---|---|
| | | | | | | Antepartum | Delivery or Postpartum | | | Complications | Wgt. | Apgar 1 & 5 Minutes | | |
| A. | Antepartum Admissions | | | | | | | | | | | | | |
| 1 | BG078331 | 24 | 3 | 2 | 34 | Preterm labor | Undelivered | Intravenous tocolytics | 2 | | | | | |
| 2 | BJ026739 | 33 | 4 | 2 | 33 | Preeclampsia, prior cesarean section | Undelivered | Aldomet, bedrest, transport to tertiary hospital | 1 | | | | | |
| 3 | BR026529 | 21 | 4 | 3 | 20 | Pyelonephritis | Undelivered | Intravenous antibiotics | 3 | | | | | |
| 4 | GP009562 | 25 | 4 | 1 | 34 | Preterm labor | Undelivered | Intravenous tocolytics | 0 | | | | | |
| 5 | JA066650 | 22 | 1 | 0 | 30 | No prenatal care, preterm labor | Undelivered | Intravenous tocolytics, steroids, transport to tertiary hospital | 0 | | | | | |
| 6 | BM47315 | 27 | 4 | 3 | 16 | 13 cm right upper quadrant mass | | Excision of dermoid cyst | 2 | | | | | |
| B. | Obstetric Deliveries | | | | | | | | | | | | | |
| 7 | SH079268 | 32 | 2 | 1 | 38 | None | Shoulder | SVD | 2 | Fractured | 4344 | 9/9 | | 2 |

Example 12   "Too Short" — The Right Way

| Initials & Hosp. # No. | Age | Gravida | Para | Diagnosis Preoperative or Admission (include size of ovarian cysts) | Treatment | Surgical Pathology Diagnosis (uterine wt. in gms.) | Complications (include blood transfusions) | Days in Hosp. |
|---|---|---|---|---|---|---|---|---|
| 29 L.P. 218515 | 32 | 3 | 2 | Left labial tear | Repair of left labial tear | | 0 | 0 |

Pass Your Oral OB/GYN Board Exam!

## Example 13   Too Many Patients Per Page

| # | Initials | Age | Gravida | Para | Problem | Diagnostic Procedures | Treatment | Results | # Visits |
|---|----------|-----|---------|------|---------|-----------------------|-----------|---------|----------|
| **Preventative Care & Health Maintenance** | | | | | | | | | |
| 174 | RA | 35 | 3 | 2012 | Annual exam<br>Polycystic ovaries | Pap, baseline mammogram<br>Cardiac profile, fasting glucose | Dietary modification | Elevated cholesterol<br>Glucose normal | 1 |
| 175 | AG | 73 | 0 | 0 | Annual exam<br>Breast CA x 1 yr, on tamoxifen<br>Atrophic vaginitis (pruritus) | Pap<br>Endometrial biopsy: atrophic | Topical estrogen | Resolution of pruritus | 3 |
| **Obesity** | | | | | | | | | |
| **Sexual Dysfunction** | | | | | | | | | |
| 176 | ME | 50 | 2 | 2004 | Decreased libido on HRT | None | Testosterone added to HRT<br>Testosterone increased | Slight improvement<br>Significant improvement | 6 |
| **Contraceptive Complications** | | | | | | | | | |
| 177 | BB | 31 | 0 | 0 | Amenorrhea on birth control pills | Pregnancy test: negative | Changed formula | Regular menses | 2 |
| 178 | VM | 63 | 5 | 5 | Postmenopausal bleeding<br>IUD perforating through cervix | IUD culture: actinomycoses<br>Endometrial biopsy: atrophic | PCN G 500 qd x 4 wk | No recurrent bleeding | 6 |
| **Genetic Problems** | | | | | | | | | |
| **Primary or Secondary Amenorrhea** | | | | | | | | | |
| 179 | JG | 33 | 2 | 0010 | 48 days from last menses<br>Requesting medical VIP | Pelvic sonogram (6-wk gestation)<br>hCG, CBS, AST, ALT: normal | Methotrexate IM<br>Misoprostol intravaginal | SAB | 4 |
| 180 | SO | 27 | 0 | 0 | Secondary amenorrhea<br>Galactorrhea | Elevated prolactin (97)<br>Pituitary MRI: microadenoma | Bromocriptine | Cyclic menses<br>Galactorrhea improved | 4 |
| 181 | LW | 25 | 0 | 0 | Post-pill amenorrhea x 8 wk | Pregnancy test: negative<br>TSH, prolactin: normal | Provera challenge | Menses | 2 |
| **Infertility** | | | | | | | | | |
| 182 | DB | 32 | 1 | 1 | Secondary infertility<br>Irregular menses | TSH = hypothyroidism | Synthroid | Cyclic menses | 2 |
| 183 | JM | 31 | 1 | 1 | Secondary infertility | HSG: no abnormalities<br>TSH, prolactin: normal<br>Semen analysis: low sperm count | None | Referral: reproductive<br>endocrinologist | 3 |
| **Endometriosis** | | | | | | | | | |
| 184 | AP | 25 | 0 | 0 | Severe dysmenorrhea<br>History of endometriosis | None | Birth control pills<br>Anaprox | Improvement | 2 |

## Example 14  Edited Version of Example 12

| # | Initials | Age | Gravida | Para | Problem | Diagnostic Procedures | Treatment | Results | # Visits |
|---|----------|-----|---------|------|---------|----------------------|-----------|---------|----------|
| 1. Patient List | | | | | | | | | |
| Preventative Care & Health Maintenance | | | | | | | | | |
| 153 | RA | 35 | 3 | 2 | Annual exam Polycystic ovary disease | Pap, baseline mammogram Cardiac profile, 2h glucose test | Dietary modification | Elevated cholesterol Glucose normal | 2 |
| 154 | AG | 73 | 0 | 0 | Annual exam Breast cancer x 1 yr, on tamoxifen Atrophic vaginitis (pruritus) | Pap Endometrial biopsy: atrophic | Topical estrogen (discussed with breast surgeon and oncologist) | Resolution of atrophy | 3 |
| Obesity - None Observed | | | | | | | | | |
| Sexual Dysfunction | | | | | | | | | |
| 155 | ME | 50 | 2 | 4 | Decreased libido on HRT | None | Testosterone added to HRT | Improvement | 6 |
| Contraceptive Complications | | | | | | | | | |
| 156 | BB | 31 | 0 | 0 | Amenorrhea on oral contraceptives | Pregnancy test: negative | Changed Estrogen from 20 mg to 30 mg | Regular menses | 2 |
| 157 | VM | 63 | 5 | 5 | Postmenopausal bleeding IUD perforating through cervix | IUD culture: actinomycoses Endometrial biopsy: atrophic | IUD removed PCN G 500 x qd 4 wk | No recurrence | 6 |
| Genetic Problems | | | | | | | | | |

Example 15   Appropriate Friedman Terminology

| # | Initials & Hosp. No. | Age | Gravida | Para | Gest. Age | Complications | | | Operative Procedures and/ or Treatment | Days in Hosp. | Newborn | | | | |
|---|---|---|---|---|---|---|---|---|---|---|---|---|---|---|---|
| | | | | | | Antepartum | Delivery or Postpartum | | | | Complications | Wgt. | Apgar 1 & 5 Minutes | Days in Hosp. |
| 127 | M.D. 175600 | 27 | 2 | 0 | 42 | Post dates | | | Cytotec cervical ripening | 4 | None | 3686 | 9/10 | 4 |
| | | | | | | Protracted active phase of dilatation | Persistent occiput posterior position | | Intrauterine pressure catheter | | | | | |
| | | | | | | | Arrest of descent | | Pitocin augmentation | | | | | |
| | | | | | | | | | Failed low vacuum extraction | | | | | |
| | | | | | | | | | Primary low transverse cesarean section | | | | | |

Example 16   Management Flow — The Wrong Way

| Initials & Hosp. # No. | Age | Gravida | Para | Gest. Age | Complications | | Days in Hosp. | Newborn | | | | |
|---|---|---|---|---|---|---|---|---|---|---|---|---|
| | | | | | Antepartum | Delivery or Postpartum | Operative Procedures and/ or Treatment | | Complications | Wgt. | Apgar 1 & 5 Minutes | Days in Hosp. |
| 11 PH001118 | 37 | 1 | 0 | 36 | Advanced maternal age, preterm, premature rupture of membranes, pregnancy-induced hypertension, Hypothyroidism | None | Synthroid, labetalol, Pitocin augmentation, low forceps delivery | 3 | None | 3156 | 7/8 | 3 |

87

## Example 17  Management Flow — The Right Way

| Initials & Hosp. # No. | Age | Gravida | Para | Diagnosis Preoperative or Admission (include size of ovarian cysts) | Treatment | Surgical Pathology Diagnosis (uterine wt. in gms.) | Complications (include blood transfusions) | Days in Hosp. |
|---|---|---|---|---|---|---|---|---|
| 62 P.C. 372236 | 45 | 2 | 2 | Abnormal uterine bleeding Endometrial thickening by vaginal sonography: 2.1 cm Stenotic cervix Office endometrial biopsy— unsuccessful | D&C | Dyssynchronous endometrium— benign | None | 0 |

Example 18  Pertinent Data "Just Right"

| # | Initials & Hosp. No. | Age | Gravida | Para | Gest. Age | Complications | | Operative Procedures and/or Treatment | Days in Hosp. | Newborn | | | |
| --- | --- | --- | --- | --- | --- | --- | --- | --- | --- | --- | --- | --- | --- |
| | | | | | | Antepartum | Delivery or Postpartum | | | Complications | Wgt. | Apgar 1 & 5 Minutes | Days in Hosp. |
| 124 | L.V. 100489 | 30 | 2 | 1 | 38 | None | Severe shoulder dystocia | Spontaneous vaginal delivery McRobert's maneuver, Suprapubic pressure, Episiotomy extension (third degree) Wood's corkscrew maneuver | 2 | None | 3912 | 8/9 | 2 |

## Chapter

# Kodachromes

The Kodachrome section was **eliminated** in 2003. I have left this chapter in, as it is too early to know for certain whether the slides are truly gone forever. Even if they are, I suggest you peruse the list, as you can easily turn them into a structured case or case of the day.

For those of the digital generation, Kodachromes are 35mm slides that can be projected onto a screen. A few isolated ones have surfaced since 2003, and they can now be projected onto the screen of laptops. They may represent any OB/GYN topic. Their role on the exam has shifted. Initially, the emphasis was on correct identification of the slide. Later, they were used as a starting point for discussion of a particular topic until they were eliminated in 2003.

Historically, there were six to nine slides: two or three each for obstetrics, gynecology, and office practice. Typically, the slides were labeled with the diagnosis; usually at least one was unknown. The labeled slides stated the diagnosis up front. Although correct identification of the unknown slide scored points, you did not lose points if you did not identify the slide correctly.

The examiners recognized that the unlabeled slides were subject to interpretation. Thus, there may have been more than one right answer for each slide. The emphasis was not on your correct identification of the Kodachrome but on the justification for your interpretation. Variable interpretations were a springboard for a variety of topics, with the examiner having less control over the agenda. Thus, the candidate had the opportunity for expression of individual, creative thinking, leading to a spontaneous discussion of various topics. On the other hand, a labeled slide defined the agenda and allowed standardization among candidates.

The set of slides changed daily. Throughout the years, however, certain slides predictably recurred. Table 1 lists those slides.

**TABLE 1**   Kodachromes on Past Exams

### I. Obstetrics

1. Monitor strips—pattern recognition, etiologies, management, indications for scalp pH
   - *Tachycardia with decreased BTBV
   - Repetitive, late, uniform deceleration
   - Sinusoidal pattern
   - *Nonreactive NST
   - Bradycardia secondary to oxytocin hyperstimulation
   - Variable decelerations with increases in baseline: types of deceleration, causes, treatment (including amnioinfusion)

2. *Face presentation through a fully dilated cervix: management (CD vs. SVD), recognition (mentum posterior vs. anterior), role of forceps vs. vacuum (contraindicated)

3. *Pedigree recognition: autosomal-recessive (cystic fibrosis, sickle cell anemia pedigree), X-linked (hemophilia pedigree): pattern of inheritance, prenatal counseling

4. Lactating breast—recognition only; usually no questions about abnormal lactation

5. Obstetric ultrasounds
   - *Duodenal atresia (double-bubble sign)
   - *Omphalocele (ultrasound or photo of newborn): differentiation from gastroschisis, association with trisomies, management (labor and newborn), prenatal counseling
   - Multifetal gestation (ultrasound of twins or five gestational sacs: recognition, zygosity, maternal and fetal risks, management [antepartum, including fetal reduction, amnio-centesis], delivery)
   - Empty gestational sac (management)
   - *Placenta previa 14 weeks EGA–labeled: definition (marginal vs. complete), accuracy of ultrasound; diagnosis, risk factors, management
   - Fetal hydrops: nonimmune (parvovirus—management of fetus, presentation in adult) vs. immune; differential diagnosis, work-up. (See also #18.)
   - Cervical length (label incompetent cervix): role of ultrasound, management cerclage (Shirodkar vs. MacDonald)

6. Fetus with anencephaly
   - AFP
   - Inheritance; recurrence rate
   - Folic acid (dose)

7. Ambiguous genitalia (management)

8. *Fetus with
   - Rocker bottom feet
   - Clenched fists
   - Micrognathia
   - Prominent occiput (Edwards' syndrome—trisomy 18)

9. *Fetus with
   - Cleft lip and palate
   - Omphalocele (Patau's syndrome, trisomy 13)

10. *Fetus with
    - *Cystic hygroma
    - *Anasarca (Turner's syndrome—45XO)

11. 14/21 balanced translocation: presentation, counseling, definition of aneuploidy, the most common types of chromosomal abnormalities, description of other presentations of Down's syndrome

12. Placenta with
    - Adherent clot on maternal surface (labeled abruption): symptoms of abruption vs. previa, risk factors, blood replacement
    - Entangled cords (See Twins, #14.)
    - Succenturiate lobe (unlabeled): management of retained placenta, significance of succenturiate lobe

13. Velamentous insertion (unlabeled): role of ultrasound, differential diagnosis of third-trimester bleeding, differentiation from vasa previa, risk factors, fetal heart rate pattern on rupture, presentation, management (APT test, Kleihauer-Betke test)

14. *Twins (photo of discordant newborns or photo of monochorionic placenta with entangled cords (see also #12): twin-to-twin transfusion (pathophysiology, which twin has the worse prognosis), zygosity

15. Photo of 3-cm dilated cervix with BBOW (see also #5): management, cerclage (technique, types), subsequent SROM at 32 wks EGA (management, antibiotics, steroids)

16. Pathology slide of chorioamnionitis: describe slide (PMNs), treatment, antibiotics (use, selection, dose, duration)

17. Pathology slide of alveolus with fat: describe slide (amniotic fluid embolus), presentation, risk factors

18. Photo of a stillborn labeled nonimmune hydrops (see also #5): discuss etiologies, treatable causes (parvovirus, tachyarrhythmias)

19. Photo of a macrosomic fetus: predisposing factors, fetal and maternal complications associated with delivery, diagnosis and prognosis of brachial plexus injury

20. Photo of a foot through the vagina (incomplete breech): management, risk of cord prolapse with frank vs. complete vs. incomplete breech, vaginal breech delivery (counseling, candidates, procedure)

21. Hysterectomy specimen with molar pregnancy: presentation, work-up, management, follow-up, karyotype

22. Photo of vulvar hematoma with 3rd-degree laceration: anatomy, management (progression to necrotizing fasciitis)

23. Intraoperative photo of inverted uterus: management

24. Photo of cellulitis cesarean section incision: presentation, management, antibiotics (selection, dose, duration)

25. Photo of a Foley catheter with hematuria after cesarean section: significance, work-up, management

26. Photo of gravid patient with exophthalmos: signs and symptoms of hyperthyroidism, maternal and fetal effects, management, treatment

## II. Gynecology

1. *Photo of procidentia: work-up and management (conservative vs. surgical); draw initial incision and course of ureters

2. *Photo of Q-tip test: technique, interpretation, management of GSUI

3. Photo of cystocele: differentiation from rectocele, office evaluation (including work-up of GSUI), conservative vs. surgical treatment, surgical technique

4. Photo of rectocele (labeled pelvic organ prolapse): differentiation from cystocele and enterocele, surgical approach with concurrent enterocele

5. *Photo of perineum of black female with Foley catheter (necrotizing fasciitis)—describe photo, differential diagnosis, work-up, management

6. KUB x-ray showing dilated loops of bowel: discuss radiographic features that distinguish SBO vs. ileus, differential diagnosis, presentation, management

7. Photo of incision with extruding loops of bowel (wound dehiscence): risk factors, intraoperative prevention, recognition, management

8. Upright KUB with air in pelvis (septic abortion): describe x-ray, differential diagnosis, prevention, management

9. KUB x-ray showing distended bowel after elective abortion (diagnosis: gas gangrene of uterus): describe x-ray, differential diagnosis, management (including decision for hysterectomy, [?BSO ?]

10. Laparoscopic photo of either IUD in cul-de-sac or perforation of fundus by IUD: presentation, complications, work-up, pathophysiology of adhesion formation

11. *Colposcopy of the cervix: adequacy of colposcopy, procedure, criteria for cone, treatment if cervical cancer IB, management (LEEP vs. cryotherapy vs. laser vs. cold-knife cone), influence of pregnancy, follow-up

12. Speculum view of large invasive cervical cancer: initial management (Pap smear? biopsy? in office?), management of bleeding, treatment depending on stage

13. Photo of a pigmented lesion on vulva (diagnosis: malignant melanoma): differential diagnosis, workup, treatment

14. *Photo of vulva with diffuse erythematous areas labeled "Paget's disease" or microscopic slide labeled "Paget's disease": identify and describe the Paget's cells, significance (underlying adenocarcinoma—where?), presentation, site of biopsy, management

15. *Ultrasound of thickened (12mm) endometrial stripe or microscopic slide of endometrial hyperplasia with atypia (unlabeled): ultrasound role and parameters, evaluation (including determination of cervical stenosis, techniques of cervical dilatation, D&C vs. office sampling), treatment with progesterone, significance of atypia, management if cancerous, staging

16. Microscopic slide labeled "granulosa cell tumor": histologic description, management in pre- vs. postmenopausal patient, role of adjuvant therapy

17. Inguinal mass: etiologies and work-up

18. *Genital chancre: differential diagnosis and work-up

19. Laparoscopic photo of ruptured tubo-ovarian abscess: presentation, differential diagnosis, management, treatment, antibiotic selection

20. Laparoscopic view of perihepatic adhesions (Fitz-Hugh-Curtis syndrome): presentation, work-up, criteria for inpatient vs. outpatient management, antibiotics, surgical vs. conservative treatment

21. *Intraoperative photo of 20cm smooth ovarian mass labeled "serous cystadenocarcinoma": preoperative work-up (role of tumor markers, CT, ultrasound), surgical approach, staging, DVT prophylaxis, adhesion prevention, recurrence, management of borderline lesions or lesions with low malignant potential

22. *Ovarian torsion: intraoperative management (conservative vs. USO)

23. Intraoperative photo of an incidental teratoma (12cm) found at cesarean section: management (cystectomy vs. oophorectomy, previous USO, mature vs. immature); describe the three cell layers

24. Gross photo of ovarian endometrioma: presentation, surgical technique of resection; describe the course of the ureter, recognition and management of ureteral obstruction intra- and postoperatively, hormone replacement

25. Ectopic pregnancy (tubal-cervical): surgical vs. medical management

26. *Laparoscopic photo of tubal ectopic pregnancy or CT scan of pelvis showing cornual ectopic pregnancy: discuss CT findings, management (depending on location, surgical vs. medical), methotrexate (mechanism, dose, side effects, efficacy, follow-up), surgery (open vs. laparoscopic, salpingectomy vs. salpingostomy), recurrence

27. Microscopic slide of tuberculosis of fallopian tube: presentation (primary infertility in Vietnamese woman), work-up, treatment

28. Rectovaginal fistula (labeled RV fistula): causes and management

29. Intraoperative photo of normal uterus, tubes and ovaries: dictate TAH, BSO

30. Hysteroscopic view of submucosal leiomyomata: describe what you see, presentation, conservative management, role of GnRH agonists, hysteroscopic management (technique, solutions, monitoring of patient)

31. Intraoperative photo of leiomyomatous uterus or hysterectomy specimen of leiomyomatous uterus: role of myomectomy, pre- and intraoperative measures to limit blood loss, conservative vs. surgical management, measures to avoid/recognize bladder and ureteral injuries, route of hysterectomy

## III. Office Practice

1. *Ultrasound of polycystic ovaries or photo of hirsute patient: diagnosis, laboratory work-up (know units), management of infertility vs. oligo- or amenorrhea, association with insulin resistance, hypertension, hyperlipidemia, role of metformin

2. Wet mount of clue cells (bacterial vaginosis)

3. Wet mount of hyphae (*Candida* sp.): treatment (resistance, recurrent)

4. *Gross or microscopic slide of vulvar dystrophy (*lichens sclerosis or squamous hyperplasia): discuss histologic features; when, how, and where to biopsy, treatment

5. Photo of pigmented skin lesion on lower extremity: discuss characteristics of benign vs. malignant lesions, biopsy technique, differential diagnosis, prognosis of melanoma, staging, treatment

6. Pediatrics
   • Vulvar lesion (hemangioma) on prepubescent female: etiology and management
   • Straddle injury
   • Labial agglutination—etiology, treatment
   • Photo of a bloody pediatric perineum (sexual assault): evaluation, specimen collection and processing, whom to notify, timing of antibiotics relative to culture result

7. Infertility
  - *Uterine leiomyomata: mechanism of infertility and management (see also gynecologic Kodachromes, page 94)
  - *Bicornuate uterus: Müllerian defects mechanism for infertility and management, associated anomalies
  - Ultrasound of transverse vaginal septum with hematometra and hematocolpos (imperforate hymen): presentation, association with endometriosis, incision (stellate vs. cruciate), differential diagnosis of primary amenorrhea in a 14-year-old girl
  - HSG of filling defect (Asherman's syndrome): infertility and management
  - Longitudinal vaginal septum (labeled): associated with what condition?—counseling issues, treatment
  - Tuberculosis of fallopian tube: see also gynecologic Kodachromes, page xx
  - Photo of perineum with vaginal agenesis: presentation, recognition, work-up, differential diagnosis, management
  - Photo of bilateral distal hydrosalpinx (labeled): work-up, treatment, success

8. Ultrasound of 8mm fetal pole without cardiac activity: work-up (serial HCGs)

9. Ultrasound or laparoscopic photo of ectopic pregnancy (labeled; see also gynecologic Kodachromes, page 94)—diagnosis (HCG, progesterone, ultrasound), counseling, medical management, methotrexate protocol, follow-up, long-term results

10. Laparoscopic view of endometriosis: diagnosis, presentation, management (intra- vs. postoperative, if patient desires vs. declines pregnancy)

11. Breast
  - *Photo of breast cyst aspiration: disposition of fluid (discard vs. cytology), recurrence management, criteria for cancer work-up, staging of breast cancer

# Case of the Day

The "case of the day" was introduced in 1994, when the ABOG eliminated the pathology microscopic slides interpretation. Thus, half of the exam entailed the Kodachromes and the case of the day. This change signaled the board's attempt to standardize the exam and introduce more objectivity to an inherently subjective format.

"Case of the day" is my term for what the board refers to as "structured cases." These are written patient management scenarios for each of the three sections. They serve as a springboard for a specific topic. The examiner cues the start with the computer mouse, and the hypothetical clinical scenarios named A, B, C, etc., appear on the screen. Each mouse click brings up a new screen or additional information or questions about the case. Unlike the questions during the case list section of the exam, ABOG and not the examiner predetermines most of these questions. The examiner does not have free rein until the end, when the computer screen displays: "Supplemental Questions by Examiner."

All the candidates from the same exam session have the same structured cases; hence the nickname "case of the day." There is a different set every day. Since 2003, when the Kodachromes were deleted, the exam has been limited to defending your case list and the case of the day. Thus, half of your test, or 30 minutes for each section, consists of the case of the day.

Like other exam components, the case of the day has also evolved. The number of the cases fluctuated from a minimum of three to as many as seven. Ultimately, ABOG decided the right number was five. Each section starts with the case of the day, then switches to defending your case list for the last half.

Since the questions are predetermined and everyone is asked the same question, the answers are predictable. As with any test, there is a bell-shaped curve of expected answers. The board has set a threshold of knowledge that must be reached in order to pass a topic. The format of the case of the day dictates standardization, yet the oral exam component also permits flexibility to go beyond the threshold or to pursue other topics.

Typically, the topic is a common management issue that the generalist frequently faces. Thus, the topics on your case list probably overlap, and so you will already be prepared to some degree. The questions require you to manage the patient systematically and to progress down the algorithm pathway, as you do every day in your practice. One of the five topics may be less common. Take comfort that your cohorts answering the same question will share your same unfamiliarity as well.

Feedback from past examiners reveals they don't even get to see the case of the day questions until the morning of the test. They collectively discuss the answers. Sometimes they don't even agree amongst themselves as to what is the correct answer. Rarely, even the examiners don't know the answers to obscure and difficult questions. They are provided guidelines by ABOG but are given latitude as to how to extract and interpret your answers, as well as the freedom to supplement with their own questions. Although only one of the pair of examiners is questioning you, both must agree with your resulting score.

The strategy for the case of the day session is straightforward. There are five sets of cases lasting 30 minutes. Thus, you should spend no longer than six minutes for each set. Since 2008, the chime to signal the halfway point at 30 minutes and to announce the switch to the case list was eliminated. However, everyone seems to complete all five cases. There is a clock in the lower corner of the laptop screen with the real time. However, you don't need to worry about the time, as the examiner should be able to keep you on pace.

Nonetheless, you don't want to dilly-dally on this session. The more questions you answer, the more points you score, and the more you dilute your wrong answers. It is not necessary to, nor does a candidate often get all answers correct. You just need to get the majority (at least 70%) correct to pass each set. Thus, if there are five questions, you can miss one set and score an overall 4/5 or 80%. However, you cannot fail two sets, as 3/5 is only 60% and will most likely result in an overall fail.

Practice is paramount to assure your success. The case of the day is clearly an example of "don't let them see you sweat." Oftentimes, the answer to the previous question is revealed in the next cued question.

Don't be rattled if you choose a different answer. Remember, you don't have to get each question correct, just the majority, so use this as an opportunity to get back on track. Don't compromise the whole set by getting unglued by one question. Besides, even if your answer is different, this doesn't necessarily mean that you missed the question. Remember, most the time, there is more than one way to "skin a cat," especially in medicine.

For example, let's say the question was, "How would you treat a patient with endometrial hyperplasia with atypia?" Let's say you chose a hysteroscopic-guided fractional D&C. But the next cued question starts out, "The patient is treated with progesterone and ..." Was your answer of D&C correct? Of course, but the test writer has to move the question along and elected to go down the left rather than your right fork of the patient management algorithm pathway. So don't get frustrated and blow the rest of the questions. Switch gears, go with the flow, recover and concentrate fully on this next question with the new information.

The case of the day is typically one of two formats. The first one is management of a specific patient from beginning to end. The other is a theme that they spin and turn. For example, the theme may be abnormal uterine bleeding in an adolescent, then in a woman of reproductive age, then in a postmenopausal woman. This section is fair and straightforward. These are not trick questions. The question is right there in black and white on the computer screen. Don't make the questions harder than they are. Chances are if you're stumped, so are your colleagues.

However, unlike on your case list, try to avoid saying that you don't know the answer to a question. The examiner will have no choice but to completely dock all the points for that sub-question, so if you guess, or at least think out loud, you can hopefully get partial credit. The worse thing that can happen is that you don't get any credit. Remember also that out of your group, somebody is going to know the answer. Again, you have nothing to lose, or rather you have everything to gain, by trying to score as many points as possible.

Just a couple of practice sessions are all that are necessary to get the hang of it. The trick is finding a review course that can simulate this aspect of the exam. In the meantime, the following tables are recollections of previous candidates.

Even if the same topic is represented, I list each candidate's questions separately, as you can appreciate how the line of questioning can be different for the same topic. The depth of exam topics reflects the candidates' recall of the topic and their line of questioning. If candidates could remember only the general topic, it is merely listed. I have often supplemented these topics with questions from the case list. It is evident how helpful reviewing the case of the day topics will be as you prepare to defend your case list. An asterisk indicates topics that have already recurred and hence have a higher likelihood of appearing on your exam.

## TABLE 1  Obstetrics

### A. Infections

1. Fifth's disease –"A prenatal patient calls, stating she was exposed to a child with Fifth's Disease"
How do you counsel her?
What labs would you order?
What are the signs/symptoms in the mother?
How would you detect if the fetus is affected?

2. Varicella—"A 24-year-old teacher comes to your office, informing you that two of her students were diagnosed with Varicella."
Discuss confirmation of exposure, immunity, VZIG, management of Varicella in pregnancy, recognition and management of pneumonia, risk to baby

3. * Herpes Simplex Virus—"A 31-year-old OG with a history of genital herpes presents to the office at 37 weeks EGA with prodromal HSV symptoms."
Describe evaluation, management, suppression, and delivery options.
In a patient with a history of HSV, but has no lesions, does that guarantee a healthy fetus at vaginal delivery?

*Case List*
What are the effects of HSV to the fetus?
What is the significance to the mom and the fetus with a primary vs. recurrent HSV?
How do you confirm infection?
How do you counsel a prenatal patient with HSV?
Do you offer suppression? If so, when and with what medication?
How does the location of a lesion affect delivery?
How does rupture of membranes affect delivery?

4. Asymptomatic bacteriuria  Discuss screening, treatment, influence on management for rest of pregnancy, labor, antibiotic selection.

5. *E. coli* urinary tract infection
Discuss management, screening urinalysis, incidence of pyelonephritis, antibiotics, suppression

6. Pyelonephritis
   a. "A 23-year-old female 29 weeks pregnant with increase frequency and urination and dysuria"
   What is her likely diagnosis?
   What are the common organisms?
   What medication would you treat her with and how long?

   b. "A 23-year-old patient 23 weeks with fever, chills, back pain, dysuria, nausea and vomiting."
   What is the most likely diagnosis?
   How would you manage her?

How would you treat this patient and for how long?
Would you give her suppression?

c. "A patient with pyelonephritis and signs of acute respiratory distress."
What is your differential diagnosis?
How would you manage her?
What are the indications for admission?
Which antibiotics would you chose?
When/how does this affect the timing of delivery?
Recognition and management of septic shock

7. Trichomonas
Discuss diagnosis, treatment depending on trimester

8. Necrotizing fasciitis—"A 24-year-old postpartum patient has a large labial mass." (See also gynecologic Kodachrome, page 94.)
Discuss initial management (exploration, packing, and antibiotics, followed by discharge).
"She returns 3 days later with a fever of 103°F."
Discuss readmission, differential diagnosis, and management.

9. HIV
a. "A patient at 10 weeks EGA is HIV positive."
Discuss labs, prognosis for mom and baby, when to begin antepartum testing, antenatal medications, timing and route of delivery, breastfeeding.

b. "An HIV positive patient in labor at 30 weeks EGA."
How would you manage her?
"If the viral load was 26,000, if CD4 count was 50"
How would you manage her?
"If membranes were ruptured?"
How would you manage her?
What are the ELISA and Western blot test?

10. Syphilis—"A patient in her first trimester presents with a painless vulvar lesion."
Discuss differential diagnosis, syphilis treatment, work-up of +RPR, penicillin-allergic patient options.

11. Hepatitis B and C—"A 25-year-old at 10 weeks EGA with a positive Hepatitis B surface antigen."
Discuss labs, management antepartum and intrapartum, prognosis for mom and baby. Discuss Hepatitis C.

12. *Group B strep (GBBS)
Discuss risk based vs. universal screening
How/when to screen, when to treat?
Which antibiotic do you use? Which antibiotic if PCN allergic?
What % of GBBS are resistant to Clindamycin or Erythromycin?
What are the concerns to the fetus?

13. Toxoplasmosis –(*Usually one of the TORCH infections appears regularly on the exam.)
a. "A 26-year-old 2G/1P veterinarian assistant at 16 weeks EGA asks about toxoplasmosis."
How do you counsel her?
What tests do you order?
"Her IgG is positive and her IgM is negative" vs. "Her IgG is negative and her IgM is positive."
How do you advise her?

b. "A patient in her first trimester of pregnancy reveals she eats raw meat. She is concerned if she has Toxoplasmosis."
How do you evaluate her?
How do you counsel her re: her risks per trimester?
"What if she doesn't eat raw meat, but has a completely indoor cat?"
Is she at risk?
How would the cat get Toxoplasmosis?
"Patient is now in her third trimester."
What are ultrasound findings to suggest in utero exposure?
What are clinical findings in the newborn characteristic of Toxoplasmosis?

c. Another candidate's line of questions on the same topic:
How is Toxoplasmosis transmitted?
What labs would you order?
How do you manage her?
What is the risk of transmission per trimester?

14. <u>Cholecystitis</u>—"A patient with a 10 weeks intrauterine pregnancy presents with fever and right upper quadrant pain"
What is your differential diagnosis? (patient ultimately has cholecystitis)
How would you work her up?
How would you treat her? (If you recommended surgery, then when?)

15. <u>Endometritis</u>—"A patient is 36 hours S/P SVD with fever 104° F. and confusion."
What is your differential diagnosis?
How would you work her up?
"The patient is diagnosed with endometritis."
What antibiotic would you treat her with and why?
What bacteria would you expect?
"Given the rapid onset of the infection, what are you concerned about??
How would you treat her now?

16. <u>SPVT</u>—"A patient runs a fever of 102° F. despite IV cephalosporin antibiotics 48 hours after a cesarean in labor."
What is your differential diagnosis and work up?
Would you continue the antibiotics?
What if two days later, she develops an 8cm right adnexal mass?
How would you treat septic thrombophlebitis?

17. <u>Chorioamnionitis</u>
What antibiotics do you use?
What organisms are you covering?
How can you decrease the infection rate when you perform a c-section on a laboring patient?
When you lift the head out of the vagina, how do you diminish contamination?
How do you decrease infection during surgery in general?

18. <u>Postpartum fever</u>
Discuss differential diagnosis (including septic pelvic vein thrombosis, necrotizing fasciitis), work-up, management, antibiotic selection, when to use heparin, when to go to OR.

19. <u>Wound infection</u>—"A patient POD #6 from a CD for CPD presents with pus draining from her incision."
Discuss work-up, management, wound care, antibiotics, threshold for re-admission.

## B. * Hypertension

1. "A 27-year-old at 29 weeks EGA with no prenatal care, past medical history significant for hypertension presents for her first visit with a BP 220/100."
   Discuss evaluation, labs, definitions of the types of hypertension, especially how to distinguish chronic hypertension from superimposed preeclampsia, medications, timing of delivery

2. "A patient at 20 weeks EGA with chronic hypertension and not on medication presents with a BP 160/110."
   Discuss labs, management, Aldomet (maternal and fetal side effects, dose, when to add a second agent), second line therapy.

3. "An 18-year-old primiparous diagnosed with preeclampsia is on magnesium sulfate and develops acute respiratory arrest."
   Discuss differential diagnosis, work-up, management, mechanism of action of MgSO4, prevention.

4. "An 18-year-old at term presents to labor and delivery with a BP 140/110, 2+ proteinuria and has a generalized seizure."
   Discuss the differential diagnosis, evaluation, management of mom and baby.
   "After infusion of MgSO4 and intrauterine resuscitation, she seizes again. Her labs reveal a creatinine 1.8 and a Mg level of 2, and her urine output has been 30cc/hour." What do you do now? (Valium/Ativan since oliguria and elevated creatinine precludes another Mg bolus)
   "The fetal heart rate drops to 60 bpm x 5 minutes." Discuss management.

5. "A patient at 26 weeks EGA presents with right upper quadrant pain."
   Discuss differential diagnosis (cholecystitis vs. preeclampsia, acute fatty liver, HELLP syndrome), work-up, management.

6. "28 weeks with hypertension, 1+ proteinuria"
   What is your differential diagnosis?
   How do you manage HELLP syndrome? (Candidate responded immediate delivery, short period of expectant management for steroids, continued expectant management.)

7. "A gravid patient with HTN near term"
   How do you evaluate HTN in pregnancy?
   What labs would you order?
   Why is the uric acid elevated?
   When do you time delivery?

8. "Patient post-op C/S for arrested labor with preeclampsia. Patient is on magnesium sulfate during the procedure and postoperatively. She begins to have a grand mal seizure in the recovery room."
   What do you do next?
   What do you treat the patient with?

9. "A patient with preeclampsia in labor and on MgSO4, starts to seize."
   How would you manage her?
   What if another bolus of MgSO4 did not work?
   How do you treat the HTN?

   *Case List*
   Criteria for severe preeclampsia, when to deliver for mild vs. severe
   Definition of severe preeclampsia, what BP would require treatment and which medications to use, when to deliver vs. observe
   Definition of gestational HTN. Chronic HTN—Which anti-hypertensive medications can you use?

How do you manage chronic HTN? What is your BP threshold to treat? Which agent would you use?

Patient with chronic HTN—What medications do you use?

Why are ACE-I contraindicated in pregnancy?

15-year-old with eclamptic seizure on PPD #5—How did you manage her?

How would you counsel her regarding future pregnancies?

Patient with chronic HTN and superimposed preeclampsia—How did you evaluate her? What counseling did you offer? What medications did you use? When do you deliver?

## C. * Diabetes

1. "A patient with GDM at 39 weeks has an U/S which shows an EFW of 4200 grams. Her cervix is long, thick, and closed."
   Discuss management, how and when you screen for GDM. Who would you screen in the first trimester? Differentiate insulin from diet controlled, White's classification, insulin management antepartum and intrapartum.

2. "A patient presents with GDM-Class A2."
   Discuss White's classification, role of HgA1C, associated congenital anomalies, medical problems associated with GDM.

3. "A 27-year-old 2G/1P at 13 weeks EGA presents for routine prenatal care. She has a history of gestational diabetes with her previous pregnancy seven years ago."
   How would you counsel her?
   Would you perform an early glucose tolerance test and/or HbA1C? What congenital abnormalities can you screen for on ultrasound?
   "Both her one and three hour glucose tolerance tests are abnormal." How do you manage her?
   "At 32 weeks an ultrasound shows an EFW of 2500g and a two-hour postprandial glucose of 160." Does this change your management? (Add insulin.)
   Discuss your plans for delivery.

4. "An obese patient with a fundal height of 46cm and a cephalic presentation presents with SROM and is dilated 3cm. Her previous baby weighed 9 pounds, 11 ounces and was delivered by forceps. Two hours later her cervix is unchanged."
   Discuss risks/benefits of CD vs. vaginal delivery, evaluation and management of macrosomia, influence of diabetes and/or history of shoulder dystocia, and/or postdates on management.

5. "Diabetic with HbA1C of 11 and obese"
   How do you calculate her ideal body weight?
   When would you order a GTT? What is your cut-off level?
   What do you want her fasting blood glucose to be?
   How do you calculate her kcal requirements?

6. "Patient presents with tachypnea and tachycardia at 20 weeks gestation."
   What is your differential diagnosis?
   What labs would your order?
   "The patient is determined to have a glucose of 420."
   How do you treat DKA?
   Are there any risks to the fetus due to DKA (in other words, any risk of IUFD)?
   What would have caused the patient to go into DKA?

   *Case List*
   How do you screen for GDM? What is your 1-hour GTT cut-off? How do you make the diagnosis based on the 3 hour GTT? How do you manage with diet? How do you instruct your patient on glucose monitoring? What are your goal glucose levels?

When do you decide to start an OHG agent? Which OHG agent do you use? When do you decide for insulin?

How do you screen for GDM? What is your 1-hour GTT cutoff? (Candidate replied 140.) "If the cut-off is 135, what does that do to the sensitivity?" What does that do to the positive predictive value? What if the patient fasts? How do you calculate the requirements of a patient's insulin? How long do you give diet a chance?

What is the White's classification? What is an A2? How would you treat her?

What would prompt you to screen in the first trimester? How do you choose between insulin vs. glyburide? When would you offer a C/S for DM vs. non-DM?

How much weight does an infant gain per week? Would you offer a C/S to a diabetic mother with EFW of 3800 at 36 weeks? (This exchange was funny because I refused to guess 300mg per week, so I told him I would do a U/S at 39 weeks and then section. He asked, What if the U/S breaks down in the entire region?" Then I said I would do Leopold's and ask the mother to compare the weight of this pregnancy with the others...He kept going, and then I said, "I would have to look up the infant weight gain per week and calculate." Then he said, "What if I just told you?" By that time, the other examiner was chuckling...LOL!! )

What are the fetal risks in terms of congenital defects? How do you counsel patients about calories and diet?

## D. Medical Complications of Pregnancy

1. Mitral stenosis with dyspnea in the second trimester
   Differentiate from aortic stenosis, and describe ante and postpartum management.

2. Renal transplant—"A patient with a history of a renal transplant presents for her first prenatal visit at 8 weeks EGA."
   Discuss counseling for termination, management, use of anti-rejection medications, influence of rising creatinine, delivery.

3. Thrombocytopenia
   a. "A patient presents at 34 weeks EGA with a platelet count of 104,000."
      Discuss differential diagnosis including differentiation of idiopathic thrombocytopenic purpura from gestational thrombocytopenia, work-up, management antepartum and intrapartum, effects on baby.

   b. "A 21-year-old G1P0 at 35 weeks with platelet count of 90,000."
      What is your differential diagnosis?
      How would you work her up?
      How would you manage her?
      Can you perform regional anesthesia in this patient?

   c. "A 35-year-old G2P1 at 20 weeks with platelet count of 50,000 and history of chronic hypertension."
      What is your differential diagnosis? What is the most likely diagnosis?
      How would you manage her if she was determined to have gestational thrombocytopenia? How would you deliver this patient at term?

4. Anemia
   a. "A 22-year-old 2G/1P at 28 weeks EGA with a Hct of 28 compared to her first trimester Hct of 37."
      Discuss differential diagnosis of anemia, work-up (including Hb electrophoresis), treatment, dose and types of iron supplementation.

b. "A 16-year-old pregnant patient has a positive sickle cell screen."
Describe the genetics, Hb electrophoresis, and management, including sickle cell crisis.

c. "A patient at 24 weeks gestation with a hemoglobin of 8.8 g/dl"
What is your differential diagnosis? How would you work her up?
"She is diagnosed with iron deficiency anemia and started on oral iron for one month. She is now at 28 weeks, but her hemoglobin is unchanged at 8.8 g/dl."
How would you treat her now? (I mentioned IV iron, so they asked me *a ton of* questions about dose/frequency/side effects, etc.!) Would you transfuse her?
"Now she is 38 weeks in labor and her hemoglobin is 8.8 g/dl."
How do you manage her? Would you transfuse her?

5. <u>Thyroid disease</u>—"A 2G/1P at 8 weeks EGA with hyperemesis and an elevated TSH"
What is your differential diagnosis? How would you evaluate for each?

"A U/S verifies an IUP. What would you expect her TSH level to be in the setting of hyperemesis?"
"Her free T4 is consistent with hypothyroidism."
How would you manage her? (Candidate chose Synthroid.)
Does Synthroid cross the placenta?
When would you recheck a T4?
What if she had hyperthyroidism?
How would you treat her? (Candidate chose PTU)
Does PTU cross the placenta?
Which crosses the placenta more, PTU or Synthroid? (*My local MFM says, "Who cares? You want the Synthroid to cross the placenta to prevent fetal hypothyroidism and mental retardation."*)

6.* <u>Thromboembolic Disease</u>—"A patient with a history of DVT"
Would you give her OCPs?
"She now presents newly pregnant"
Discuss genetic causes, management antepartum, intrapartum   and postpartum, heparin and low molecular weight heparin (mechanism of action, dose, monitoring, pros/cons), neonatal risks, management subsequent pregnancies.

# E. Intraterine Growth Restriction (IUGR)

a. "33 weeks by LMP, +urine pregnancy test, late prenatal care, U/S = 28 weeks EGA"
How would you evaluate her?
How would you manage her?
What is the difference between symmetric vs. asymmetric IUGR?
What are causes for each?

b. "Patient comes in at 34 weeks with IUGR."
Discuss antenatal testing
How would you manage the pregnancy? Inpatient? Outpatient?
S/D ratio of umbilical Dopplers. What does it mean?
When do you decide to deliver?
Discussion of asymmetric vs. symmetric IUGR—Causes, risks, management
Other candidates had isoimmunization questions and had to follow MCA Dopplers and had to explain the algorithm about checking the father's blood type, etc.

c. "A patient at 32 weeks EGA by LMP and early ultrasound now has an ultrasound measuring 28 weeks."
Differentiate asymmetric from symmetric IUGR, discuss etiologies and management.

*Case List*
How do you define asymmetric vs. symmetric IUGR?
What are causes of each?
How would you monitor her antenatally?

## F. Genetics

1. <u>Advanced maternal age</u>
   a. "A 34-year-old 0G on OCPs for 15 years comes for preconception counseling."
   Describe preconception counseling, first-trimester genetic counseling, and prenatal risk factors, amniocentesis vs. CVS.

   b. AMA and aneuploidy risks – First vs. second trimester screen, CVS vs. amniocentesis

2. <u>Preconception counseling</u>—"A 24-year-old who has a nephew with cystic fibrosis comes for preconception counseling."
   Describe inheritance patterns, risk of disease, antenatal testing, and presentation of newborn.

3. <u>Down's Syndrome</u>—"An anatomic screening U/S at 18 weeks reports nuchal thickening."
   Discuss differential diagnosis, ultrasound markers, Down's syndrome-inheritance, phenotype, medical complications to baby, screening, termination counseling and technique, management during pregnancy.

4. <u>Maternal serum screening</u>
   Discuss components of triple/quadruple markers, significance, management if elevated vs. decreased, sensitivity/specificity.

## G. Emergencies

1. *<u>VBAC</u> – "A 26-year-old 2G/1P prior CD in labor has sudden vaginal bleeding, fetal bradycardia, and loss of fetal station."
   Describe diagnosis, management, and prevention, and whether a candidate for VBAC counseling.

2. * <u>Abruption</u>
   a. "At 36 weeks EGA, no fetal movement has been detected for one month. Ultrasound confirms IUFD in a transverse lie, PT and PTT are elevated twofold, the platelet count is 70,000, fibrinogen is decreased, and fibrin split products are elevated."
   Describe the work-up, management (cryoprecipitate vs. FFP, type of delivery, transverse vs. vertical CD), and complications (persistent postoperative fever in spite of ATBs).

   b. "A patient at 32 weeks EGA with contractions and vaginal bleeding"
   What is your differential diagnosis? (Patient ended up having an abruption.)
   When would you move to delivery vs. observation?

   c. "A 23-year-old patient at 23 weeks EGA is complaining of abdominal pain. She is positive for cocaine. There are no fetal heart tones auscultated and she oozing from incision site (not clear what/when this incision was made)."
   How would you manage the patient?
   Describe the various types of blood products and how would you use them?

   d. "A patient at 32 weeks EGA is rear ended in a motor vehicle accident. She was wearing her seat belt and did not sustain obvious abdominal trauma. She complains of shoulder pain. Her vital signs are stable."
   Discuss evaluation, labs (including Kleihauer-Behtke, aPTT coagulation panel), role of U/S, fetal monitoring (duration). "A CD is performed for fetal distress, and blood is in the abdomen." Discuss management, expected injuries.

e. "A patient presents at 28 wks EGA with heavy vaginal bleeding and contractions every two minutes."
Discuss differential diagnosis, work-up, evaluation.
"If the diagnosis is IUFD noted on U/S, does this change your diagnosis?"
Discuss abruption, DIC, labs (including Kleihauer-Betke), management, blood component therapy, route of delivery.

3. Previa
a. "A 35-year-old 3G/2P with 2 prior CDs and a known complete placenta previa presents with vaginal bleeding."
Discuss counseling, timing of delivery, pre-op prep, autologous blood donation, type of skin incision.

b. "A patient with three prior CDs has a placenta previa."
Discuss counseling, timing of delivery, pre-op prep, autologous blood donation, type of skin incision.

c. "A patient at 28 weeks EGA with contractions and vaginal bleeding"
What is your differential diagnosis? (Patient ended up having a placenta previa.)
How would you manage her if she had a complete placenta previa?
When would you deliver her?

d. "A patient at 28 weeks EGA with contractions and vaginal bleeding"
What is your differential diagnosis? (Patient ended up having a vasa previa)
How would you manage her: inpatient or outpatient?
When would you deliver her?

e. "A patient with a known placenta previa with a recent bleed, but is currently no longer bleeding?"
What are your concerns?
"Her Hb is 7.5 and her vital signs are stable"
Would you transfuse her?
How do you counsel her on a blood transfusion?

*Case List*
How to evaluate documentation of placentation?
What is your delivery plan if you suspect an accreta?
Discuss management, type of uterine incision, risk, recognition, and management of placenta accreta.

4. Embolism
a. "On POD 3 after primary cesarean delivery for failed induction for preeclampsia, a patient has tachypnea, pulse oximeter 88 and PaO2 76, and dyspnea. She is afebrile."
Discuss work-up, invasive monitoring, and treatment.

b. "A 25 year-old G2P1 undergoing routine cesarean delivery has sudden onset of dyspnea and cardiorespiratory arrest."
What is your differential diagnosis?
How would you evaluate and manage her?
Assuming she survives a code, what labs would you be concerned about?

5. Neonatal resuscitation—"A 26-year-old 2G/1P delivers the second twin without respiratory effort."
Discuss the differential diagnosis (answer: respiratory depression secondary to maternal narcotics) and management.

6. *Postpartum hemorrhage
   a. "Extension of uterine incision at cesarean section ultimately leads to cesarean hysterectomy."
   Describe management, prevention, anatomy, and supracervical hysterectomy vs. TAH.

   b. Postpartum hemorrhage
   Work-up, medical management (which drug, mechanism of action, dosing, frequency, side effects, contraindications), embolization surgical management (uterine artery ligation, B-Lynch suture, hemostatic square sutures, hypogastric artery ligation, cesarean hysterectomy).

   c. "Patient who is postpartum with a mass hanging out of vagina"
   What is your differential diagnosis?
   "Patient has an uterine inversion with an intact placenta"
   Do you remove the placenta?
   How do you evaluate/treat the patient? (They continued to ask what else until you took her to the OR for exploratory laparotomy, etc.)

7. Maternal hypotension: "A 22-year-old 1G/0P becomes hypotensive after placement of an epidural in labor."
   Discuss recognition, management (maternal and fetal), and prevention.

8. Post partum complications
   a. "Postpartum with a mass at introitus"
   What is your differential diagnosis? (This was a hematoma.)
   How would you treat her? What else, what else? (Ended up referring to interventional radiologist to stop the hemorrhage.)

   b. "Post partum hemorrhage"
   What is your differential diagnosis?
   How do you manage her? (This was a retained placenta, ?accreta)
   What else do you do? (Up to exploratory laparotomy/hysterectomy/ hypogastric artery ligation/UAE as option.)
   "Patient started oozing as you made the abdominal incision"
   What is your differential diagnosis? (Patient had DIC.)
   How do you evaluate her?
   How do you treat her?

   c. "Breakdown of episiotomy"
   What is your differential diagnosis?
   What are the risk factors for this?
   How would you treat her?
   Would you use antibiotics? If so, which ones?
   When to repair?

9. Cord Prolapse—"A multigravida at term gestation is 8cm in active labor. On exam you palpate an umbilical cord on the side/next to the fetal head. It is not prolapsed. The fetal heart tracing is reassuring."
   How would you manage her if the membranes are intact?
   How would you manage her if the membranes are ruptured?
   How would you manage her if the cord prolapses?

10. *Shoulder Dystocia
    a. "A patient at 36 weeks EGA is measuring 40cm on her fundal height."
    What is your differential diagnosis?
    How would you work her up?
    "Her ultrasound shows a normal AFI and an EFW of 4500 gm."
    What is the error range for ultrasound?

How does this compare to the obstetrician's estimate?
How do you manage her now?
"The patient has gestational diabetes."
Would you induce her"
"The patient has had a previous shoulder dystocia."
Would you induce her?
When would you offer a CD?

b. Candidate could not remember specifics, but topic was shoulder dystocia. Discuss management all the way to Zavanelli maneuver, difference between Duchenne's and Klumpke's palsy, discuss pelvimetry.

*Case List*

1. Maneuvers, really grilled on exactly how I would deliver the posterior arm. Also, they then asked if the baby had a brachial plexus injury. Would I advise her to deliver vaginally next time? I said I would counsel her that either CD or VD would be appropriate depending on her preference. They pressed me on what I would recommend, and I said VD. They asked what if there was a clavicular injury, would that change my recommendation? I said no. They asked me if the baby broke its humerus if that would change my recommendation? I said no. Who knows if it was the right answer!

2. Maneuvers, including corkscrew (I showed off and mentioned both Wood's and Rubin's), posterior arm, Gaskin.

3. Can you predict shoulder dystocia? What are the maneuvers and the risks associated with shoulder dystocia?

11.* Breech

a. "A term multigravida presents with a frank breech presentation with delivery imminent"
What are her anesthesia options?
Describe how you would deliver her.
How would you manage nuchal arms?
How could you prevent nuchal arms?
How do you manage an entrapped head?

b. "Breech presentation in active labor with breech crowning at introitus, vaginal delivery is inevitable."
Discuss management, steps of a vaginal breech delivery, prevention, version (singleton vs. second twin, technique, monitoring, tocolytics, success), risks to mom and baby.

c. "A 22-year-old 2G/1P presents at 36 weeks EGA with a breech presentation. Her previous delivery was vaginal. The EFW is 3700 gm."
Discuss counseling about delivery options, risks, criteria for vaginal delivery, version, pelvimetry.

d. "Term vaginal breech, baby has delivered to the umbilicus, you encounter nuchal arms."
What do you do?
Describe your technique to effect delivery.
How do you apply Piper's forceps?

e. "A patient presents at full dilation with a breech."
How do you deliver her?
What are risk factors for breech? (Went on to talk about the steps in breech delivery down to Duhrssen's incisions. Also discussed ECV.)

*Case List*
1. Technique and contraindications for external cephalic version (ECV)
2. Technique for vaginal breech delivery, including Piper's forceps
3. How do you counsel a patient on ECV?
4. The discussion started with, "I see you have a failed external cephalic version on your case list."
   How do you counsel your patients regarding external cephalic version?
   What do you tell them?
   What are the indications?
   What's your percentage of success and your failure rate?
   Where do you do the version?
   Do you give a tocolytic?
   Why don't you give anesthesia?
   When do you do the version?
   What are the contraindications to version?
   What's your fluid level cut-off for doing the version?
   Describe your technique.
5. Discussed vaginal breech extraction. I got grilled hard on this. The examiner interrupted me frequently and wanted to know precise details: How to prevent nuchal arms, where to put your hands, when to cut episiotomy. Then it went on to, "You are successful in a version and the baby turned, but shows up to labor and delivery with the breech coming out of the introitus. She's crowning and you can't push her back up. Basically, you are forced to deliver the breech vaginally. Describe the maneuvers They let me deliver the breech and did not pump me on anything else, but one candidate got nuchal arms, and another candidate had head entrapment and had to place Piper's forceps and they asked how do you apply them and how do you pull

12. <u>Malpresentation</u>—"A multigravida at term gestation in active labor. On exam you palpate a fetal arm. The fetal heart tracing is reassuring."
    How would you manage her?
    "A 16-year-old nulliparous at term and 5cm with a brow presentation"
    How would you evaluate her?
    How would you counsel her?
    How would you manage her?
    Are there any fetal situations that would predispose to brow presentation?
    "What if this 16-year-old at 5cm was noted to have a mentum   presentation?"
    How would you evaluate her?
    How would you counsel her?
    How would you manage her?
    "What if this 16-year-old at 5cm was noted to have a transverse presentation?"
    What else do you want to know about the lie of the fetus?
    How would you evaluate her?
    How would you counsel her?
    How would you manage her?
    What kind of incision would you make?
    How do you counsel the patient re: future pregnancies?

13. <u>Vulvar hematoma</u>—"A 21-year-old 1G/0P who had a low forceps delivery 20 minutes ago without severe vulvar/vaginal pain"
    Discuss differential diagnosis. (Answer: vaginal hematoma.) Evaluation (type and cross, H/H, clot hold), management non-expanding vs. expanding, ligation and packing unsuccessful and patient becomes hemodynamically unstable. What is blood supply to vulva and vagina? Patient taken to OR.
    Management (Answer: laparotomy, expanding broad ligament hematoma).

## H. Labor and Induction/Augmentation

1. Prolonged second stage of labor—"A patient has been pushing in second stage of labor for an hour. The head is at zero-station with an occipit-posterior-position."
Draw the Friedman curve, rate of Pitocin, management (forceps vs. vacuum vs. CD), 4th degree episiotomy management.

2. CPD—"A 1G/0P presents with prominent spines, and a narrow arch arrests at −1 station."

3. Dysfunctional labor: "A patient in labor has arrested at 6cm."
Discuss diagnosis of dilation arrest, role of an IUPC, Pitocin (mechanism of action, dose, side effects, management, complications).

4. Postdates and macrosomia
Define postdates vs. post-term, influence of size and gestation, timing of induction, Bishop's score (components, calculation, association with inductibility), methods of cervical ripening, influence of macrosomia and/or GDM on mode of delivery.

5. "3 of 5 of the cases were about induction of labor:
   1. for a mid-trimester loss (approximately 16-18 weeks)
   2. For a 34-week gestation with severe preeclampsia with a cervical exam closed/thick.
   3. For a 42-week gestation with a cervical exam closed/thick.

   *Case List*
   Discussed labor induction: indications, methods, risks/benefits of each method.
   Labor induction vs. CD f or macrosomia. What EFW to offer CD? What if the patient is diabetic?
   Do you offer elective inductions? When? What is the evidence for inducing for macrosomia?
   What agents do you use for cervical ripening? What is their mechanism of action?
   Pitocin—mechanism of action, dosing, side effects, contraindications, management of tachystole, hyperstimulation
   Do you use IUPCs? What are the units of measurement? How do you interpret the readings?

## I.* Incompetent Cervix, Preterm Labor, Preterm Delivery

1. Preterm labor
   a. "A 32-year-old 2G/1P with a history of preterm delivery at 36 weeks presents at 32 weeks with contractions every 4 minutes. Her cervix is long, thick, and closed." Discuss diagnosis, etiologies, and management (including pulmonary edema).

   b. "A patient at 28 weeks EGA present with regular contractions and cervix dilated to 3cm." Work-up (including fetal fibronectin), management (tocolytics, steroids, antibiotics.

2. PPROM:
   a. "A patient at 18/26/35 weeks EGA presents with obvious ROM."
   Discuss confirmation, management, role of antenatal steroids, GBBS prophylaxis, assessment of fetal lung maturity, differentiation between chorioamnionitis and abruption.

   b. PROM—"1G/0P at 36 weeks EGA with PROM"
   Discuss management (induction vs. expectant, influence of EGA), steroids, antibiotics

3. Incompetent cervix
   a. "29 y/o G1P0 with findings on sonogram at 16 weeks of 1cm cervix and funneling" How do you counsel management and treatment options?

Cerclage vs. no cerclage?
How do you counsel her on the risks benefits percentages of each?
What type of cerclage would you perform?
What suture material do you use?
"Now a G2P1 with a prior 34-week delivery is 22 weeks pregnant with cervical findings of 1cm dilated and 100% effaced"
What do you tell her?
How do you manage the pregnancy ?
When do you administer 17-OH progesterone at what gestational age?
What are the risks/benefits of 17-OH progesterone?

b. "A patient at 8 weeks EGA has a history of two prior second-trimester losses."
Describe the work-up of recurrent losses, role of MRI vs. ultrasound and cerclage.

c. "A 38-year-old G1P0 at 16 weeks with a cervical length of 2.5cm"
What is your differential diagnosis?
How do you evaluate and manage?
How do you counsel patient?

d. "A 27-year-old with prior preterm births at 22 weeks with cervical length of 1.7cm and funneling, on L&D"
What is your differential diagnosis?
How do you evaluate and manage?
How do you counsel the patient?

e. " A patient at 20 weeks EGA with cervical length of 1.5cm with contractions"
How do you evaluate her?
How do you manage her?
"Patient is now 22 weeks EGA with cervical length of 1cm."
How do you evaluate her?
How do you manage her?

*Case List*
1. What is the role of 17-OH progesterone, ultrasounds for cervical length, and fetal fibronectin? What is the mechanism of action for each drug/test? When do you order these tests or medications?
2. How does gestational age affect your management of PROM? How do you diagnose chorioamnionitis? What organisms would you expect? What antibiotics would you use?
3. How do you check for ruptured membranes? What does nitrazine paper tell you? What is ferning? Does anything else cause ferning?
4. Preterm labor management—What tocolytic do you use ? What are the other options/risks/benefits? How does magnesium sulfate work? How does it prevent seizures? If she continues to contract, what do you do? Do you add another agent?
5. Finding of short cervix on second trimester sonogram, with progressive shortening. When to do cerclage? What if she had prior 32-week delivery, then what treatment would you recommend?

## J. Non-reassuring FHR

a. "Second stage of labor with prolonged decelerations with pushing, +1 station"
How do you manage?
"The decelerations resolve with patient not pushing."
How do you manage?
"Different patient: Late active phase, rapidly progressive labor, recurrent late decelerations with moderate variability and accelerations with scalp stimulation"
How do you manage?

"Different patient: Late second stage, nulliparous, +3 station with recurrent variable decelerations"
How do you manage?

b. FHR interpretation—See Chapter 6, Kodachromes, Table 1, Obstetrics: 1. Monitor strips.

## K. Operative vaginal delivery

*Case List*
1. Indications for a vacuum assisted delivery
2. When is vacuum contraindicated? How do you place the vacuum? Do you have a pressure gauge? What are the units for your pressure gauge? How do you know how much pressure to use?
3. Discussed forceps and vacuum: when to do forceps, exactly what blades to use, fetal station, how to determine the application is correct and symmetrical.

## L. Multifetal pregnancy

1. <u>Twins</u>

a. "A 33-year-old primiparous presents with 32 weeks EGA twins. An ultrasound for growth shows a discordance."
Discuss monitoring growth, causes for discordance, zygosity, placentation, twin-to-twin transfusion.

b. Twins
How to determine chorionicity and amniocity, compare risks for MC vs. DC, how to diagnose and manage twin-to-twin transfusion syndrome.

## M. Isoimmunization

a. <u>Hydrops</u>—"G2P1 with fetal hydrops at 28 weeks"
What is your differential diagnosis? Would you order any labs? If so, which ones?
"Okay, it's nonimmune hydrops"
How do you evaluate fetus? What are risks to mother?

b. "A patient at 14 weeks EGA has a positive Coombs' test."
Discuss work-up, direct/indirect Coombs'.

## N. Adnexal mass

a. "A 23-year-old G1P0 at 10 weeks with 8cm simple adnexal mass"
What is your differential diagnosis?
How would you work her up?
How would you manage her?
"If she then presents at 20 weeks with acute abdominal pain"
What is your differential diagnosis?
How would you manage her?

b. "A 26-year-old G2 P1 at 15 weeks gestation with 10 cm adnexal mass"
What is your differential diagnosis?
How would you evaluate her?
How would you manage her?

c. "A 12cm adrenal mass is discovered during a CD."
Management (USO-dysgerminoma): Would you stage her? What if the other ovary also had a 6cm mass?

d. Ovarian mass at 18 wks EGA (teratoma vs. luteoma)

## O. Abnormal Pap Smear

    a. "A patient at 15 weeks gestation with HSIL Pap smear"
        How would you counsel her?
        How would you manage her?

    b. "Patient with extensive vulvar and cervical condyloma at 35 weeks, in for her first prenatal visit"
        How do you counsel her about risks and treatment options?

    c. "A prenatal patient at 10 weeks gestation with HGSIL Pap smear"
        How would you manage her?
        "The colposcopy shows CIN III"
        How would you manage her?
        "An OB patient at 35 weeks with multiple cervical and vulvar condylomata"
        How would you manage her?
        How would you treat her?
        Does she need a CD?

## P. Intrauterine Fetal Demise (IUFD)

    a. "Stillbirth at 16 weeks, 26 weeks, 36 weeks"
        How do you evaluate stillbirth at each gestational age?

    b. "A 20-year-old with a 21 week IUFD"
    What is your differential diagnosis?
    What are the treatment options and risk/benefits of each?
    How would you counsel the patient about options of treatment

## Q. Breast Disease

    a. "8 weeks PP, breast feeding patient with severe dyspareunia"
        What is your differential diagnosis?
        What is your most likely diagnosis?
        "Her episiotomy is intact and non-infected. What is the most likely diagnosis now? (Candidate replied atrophy secondary to breastfeeding.)
        How would you treat her?
        How would you counsel the patient?
        "Then they tried to convince me to make the patient stop breast feeding so she could get better. . . but I did not."

    b. "A women presents in pregnancy with a breast lump."
        What is your differential diagnosis?
        How would you evaluate her?
        How would you manage if she were 20 weeks pregnant?
        How would you manage if she were 30 weeks pregnant?

## R. Other

  1. Radiation exposure—"Radiation exposure at 8 weeks EGA."
      Discuss the effects of radiation, management.

  2. Flying—"Patient inquiring if she can fly during pregnancy."
      Discuss risks, contraindications, effect of non-pressurized cabins.

  3. Exercise—"Patient inquiring if she can exercise during pregnancy."
      Discuss types of exercise, impact on pregnancy, risks.

4. <u>Hyperemesis</u>—"Patient in first trimester presents with nausea, vomiting, and abdominal pain."
  Discuss differential diagnosis, work-up, management.

5. <u>Circumcision</u>
  Discuss how you counsel the parent, blood supply to the penis, pros/cons for local anesthetic, technique, complications.

6. <u>Gastroschesis vs. Omphalocele (see also Kodachromes, Chapter 6)</u>
  What would you expect her quadruple screen to be for each?
  Which is associated with chromosomal abnormalities?
  What are the ultrasound findings?
  When would you deliver her?
  What is the recommended route of delivery for each?

7. <u>Cerebral palsy</u> and neonatal encephalopathy
  Differential diagnosis
  Diagnostic criteria for hypoxic encephalopathy

8. <u>Fetal alcohol syndrome</u>—"Patient with alcohol use"
  How do you screen, and what is a safe alcohol consumption during pregnancy?
  What are the features of fetal alcohol syndrome?
  How do you manage an alcoholic patient during labor and postpartum?

9. <u>Polysubstance abuse</u> in pregnancy
  Effect on mother and fetus. What other things do you consider? (Which led to a discussion on domestic abuse and STDs. I was asked if I do a routine screen for domestic abuse.)

10. <u>Obesity</u> and pregnancy
  (I have a lot of OB patients with BMIs >35) Maternal risks, fetal risks, risks of labor dystocia, C/S. I went into detail regarding anesthesia consultation, surgical exposure, wound closure, modified Smead- Jones, suture type, prophylactic antibiotics, indications for a second antibiotic, post comps, early ambulation, DVT prophylaxis, IS, and risks of obesity and associated co-morbidities

---

## TABLE 2   Gynecology

### A. Oncology

1.*<u>Abnormal Pap smears</u>
  a. "A 26-year-old has a ASCUS Pap smear and no prior abnormal Pap smears."
    What options are there to address this pap smear?
    "A different patient has a biopsy proven CIN 1."
    How do you follow her?

  b. "A patient with adenocarcinoma-in-situ on colposcopic-directed biopsy"
    How would you manage her?
    What do you do if her cold knife cone margins are positive?

  c. "A PMP patient has a Pap smear with AGUS."
    Discuss work-up, causes, management

*Case List*
1. Management of abnormal Pap smears per age group
2. Patient had a CKC (cold knife conization).
3. How do you decide to do a LEEP vs. a CKC?
4. How do you follow a patient with CIN III on LEEP with positive margins?
5. How do you counsel that patient?

2. <u>Cervical cancer</u>—"A 30-year-old who underwent supracervical hysterectomy for postpartum hemorrhage four years ago presents with profuse vaginal discharge and spotting."
Discuss work-up, trachelectomy technique, colposcopy, site of biopsy, cervical cancer staging.

3. *<u>Adnexal mass</u>
    a. "A 23-year-old female with a history of endometriosis has an 7cm complex adnexal mass."
    What is your differential diagnosis?
    How would you work her up?
    What ultrasound features are suggestive of malignancy vs. benign?
    What are the ultrasound features of a dermoid?
    What is your recommended surgical technique for removal?
    How would your approach differ if it is now a 55-year-old with a 7cm complex adnexal mass?

    b. "A 30-year-old with an adnexal mass"
    What is your differential diagnosis?
    How would you evaluate her?
    Would you perform any imaging studies?
    What ultrasound features are suggestive of malignancy vs. benign?
    "In the OR, a frozen section shows a mucinous LMP tumor"
    Would you stage her?
    How would you stage her?
    Would you do anything else? (Candidate chose an appendectomy.)

    c. "An asymptomatic patient ?age with a 6cm endometrioma who desires future fertility"
    How do you work her up?
    "Patient is now premenopausal with a simple cyst"
    Would you take her to the OR?

    d. "A 12-year-old patient with expanding abdominal girth"
    What is your differential diagnosis?
    What is the most likely diagnosis?
    How do you evaluate her?
    What imaging and laboratory evaluation, tumor markers?
    (Diagnosis: dysgerminoma)
    How would you manage her?
    Would you stage her? If so how?
    What would necessitate a TAH/BSO in a 12-year-old female?

    e. "A 65-year-old with a 5cm cystic adnexal mass"
    What is your differential diagnosis?
    What is the most likely diagnosis?
    How would you work her up?
    What imaging and laboratory evaluation, tumor markers?
    Discuss her treatment options: laparoscopy vs. open surgery—how do you decide?

    f. "A 17-year-old/45-year-old/72-year-old is referred to you for a 8cm adnexal mass."
Discuss differential diagnosis, work-up, tumor markers, management, imaging features characteristic for benign vs. malignant, treatment for borderline vs. malignant.

    g. "An 18-year-old 0G with left lower quadrant pain, negative ßhCG, and 6cm ovarian cyst on ultrasound."
Discuss differential diagnosis, work-up, management.

## 4. Ovarian Cancer

    a. "A patient presents for her annual exam and updates you that her mother has ovarian CA."
Discuss indications, counseling for BRCA1, 2 testing, counseling depending on results, inheritance.

    b. "A 60-year-old with an 8cm pelvic mass has hydrothorax and ascites."
Discuss differential diagnosis, tumor markers, Meigs syndrome, work-up, treatment.

    c. "An 18-year-old with a dysgerminoma"
Discuss likelihood of malignancy, bilateral, recurrence risk, management of recurrence, tumor markers, fertility issues, treatment

## 5. Endometrial Cancer

*Case List*

Patient underwent D&C hysteroscopy for PMPB, and diagnosis was moderately differentiated adenocarcinoma. They used this case to ask about management of abnormal pathology on endometrium.
How would you manage if premenopausal women with hyperplasia no atypia?
How would you manage if premenopausal women with hyperplasia with atypia?
How would you manage if postmenopausal women with hyperplasia no atypia?
How would you manage if postmenopausal women with hyperplasia with atypia?
What progestin do you usually give? (what are the other options?)
How do you follow?

## 6. Vulva

    a. VIN III

        i. "A 19-year-old/32-year-old/65-year-old presents with vulvar itching and white patches on her vulva."
Differential diagnoses of vulvar pruritus, work-up, colposcopy (technique, site of biopsy), treatment.

        ii. "A 64-year-old with two reddish ulcerated lesions on vulva. Asymptomatic."
What is your differential diagnosis?
How would you evaluate her?
Would your evaluation differ if she were 32 years old? (Candidate responded she would biopsy **both**.)
"The diagnosis is VIN 3."
What are her treatment options?
Which one would YOU recommend? (Candidate responded excision.)
Describe your surgical technique.
Her margins are positive. Now what?

*Case List*

A 77-year-old patient with VIN recurrent. Candidate performed a wide local incision. What were other treatment options?

b. Vulvar Paget's Disease

   i. "A 60+-year-old has erythema and an ulcerative lesion on her vulva."
What is your differential diagnosis?
How would you evaluate each?
"A biopsy reveals Paget's disease. What is the next step? (*None of the candidates
I talked with listed Paget's in their differential.*)
How would you treat her? (Don't forget to look for underlying adenocarcinoma
elsewhere, such as breast, colon, etc.)
"If the edges of your vulvectomy cannot be approximated, then how will you
manage her? (Of course, no consultant—plastic surgeon, general surgeon, nor
oncologist—was available. This candidate knew she would need a flap, but the
examiner responded, "Where will you get your flap from?"
How will you monitor the patient in the future?
How will you treat a local recurrence?

   ii. "Pink/white lesion on vulva in a postmenopausal vs. young female"
Discuss differential diagnosis, selection of site for biopsy (reveals Paget's disease),
treatment: wide local excision vs. vulvectomy, how to decide if lymph node sampling is necessary.

7. Gestational Trophoblastic Disease

   a. GTD—"Patient develops pulmonary edema after evacuation; trophoblastic embolus with ARDS.
Discuss management.

   b. Molar pregnancy

      i. "Patient with a D&C for a molar pregnancy"
What would you do if she returns to the office with bleeding?
You now see a 3cm mass in the fornix. What is your differential diagnosis?
Would you biopsy her in the office? (Feedback from those who did: The
patient hemorrhaged.)
Your biopsy shows choriocarcinoma. How would you manage her?

      ii. "A 20-year-old at 12 weeks with nausea and vomiting"
What is your differential diagnosis?
How would you work her up?
"Ultrasound shows S/D discrepancy and snow storm appearance."
Diagnosis = molar pregnancy
How would you manage her?
What studies are needed, pre-op prep, Rh immunoprophylaxis?

## B. Emergencies

1. * Ectopic pregnancy

   a. "A 22-year-old 0G presents with right lower abdominal pain. Her LMP was
6 weeks ago and she had been using the rhythm method for contraception."
Discuss differential diagnosis, work-up, management: medical vs. surgical
(laparotomy vs. laparoscopy, salpingectomy vs. salpingostomy). If etiology was
a torsion: twist or untwist?

   b. "A patient who underwent a linear salpingostomy for an ectopic pregnancy presents 7 days later with a HCG titer of 560. Five days later, the HCG titer is 1120."
Discuss differential diagnosis, work-up, methotrexate (mechanism of action,
contraindications, dose, monitoring, side effects).

   c. "A 22-year-old presents to your office with a positive HCG, hypotensive, HR 140
and vaginal bleeding and pelvic pain."

What is your differential diagnosis?
How would you evaluate her
How would you do her surgery (laparoscopy vs. laparotomy)?
"It is a ruptured interstitial pregnancy."
How would you manage?

d. "An 18-year-old with history of infertility and 7 weeks of amenorrhea presents with spotting, and you see a bulge, mass on her cervix"
What is your differential diagnosis?
How do you evaluate her?
How do you manage a cervical ectopic pregnancy? Surgical? Medical?

e. "A young woman with 7 weeks of amenorrhea and vaginal bleeding"
What is your differential diagnosis?
How do you evaluate?
"Ultrasound demonstrates an ectopic pregnancy."
How do you manage her?
What is the dose of methotrexate (MTX)?
What is MTX's mechanism of action?
What are the side effects of MTX?
What are the indications for medical therapy vs. surgical therapy?
When do you retreat or give a second dose?
Have you ever administered a second dose?

*Case List*
1. What are indications for surgical management for an ectopic pregnancy?
2. Salpingectomy vs. salpingotomy (all different case scenarios).
What are the contraindications and indications of each, risks/benefits
3. Methotrexate—mechanism of action, candidates, risks, benefits, contraindications, counseling, dosing, monitoring, complications
4. How do you perform a wedge resection?
How would you counsel the patient regarding her risk of ectopic pregnancy in the future after a wedge resection?
In what situation would you do a hysterectomy?
5. How would you counsel the patient regarding her risk of ectopic pregnancy in the future?

2. Torsion—" A 16-year-old female G0P0 with acute pelvic/ lower abdominal pain"
What is your differential diagnosis?
How would you work her up?
"Patient had a 15cm paratubal cyst with adnexal torsion."
How would you manage her?

## C. Surgical Complications

1. *Wound Healing Complications
   a.* Dehiscence
      i. "You are called by the nurse to see a patient who had an exploratory laparotomy two days ago. You notice the dressing saturated with a serosanguinous drainage."
      Discuss management, delineate seroma vs. dehiscence vs. evisceration, or management, suture selection and closure.

      ii. "A patient is POD #? from a TAH and is noted to have copious fluid draining from her incision."
      What is your differential diagnosis? (This candidate listed dehiscence, seroma, and a bladder injury.)

How would you evaluate each?
How would you manage each?

    iii. "A 40-year-old female who is 7 days S/P TAH with midline incision presents with temperature of 101° F. and drainage from her incision."
What is your differential diagnosis?
How do you manage?
What if you find a 3cm fascial defect on opening the wound?
How would you manage?

    iv. "Case of a post-op wound dehiscence S/P TAH/BSO. Patient was a diabetic and obese. Eventually found patient to have fascial dehiscence.

    v. "An obese lady has a serous discharge from her incision 6 days after a hysterectomy."
What is the most likely cause?
When and in whom will you perform secondary closure?
When will you leave a wound open to close by secondary intention?

b. Hernia
Incisional hernia, umbilical hernia
Discuss recognition, work-up, management, principles of hernia repair including decision making to place a graft, graft selection, and surgical technique, management if need to excise through mesh.

c. Necrotizing fasciitis (See Office R, Vulvar disease page 146.)

d. "A patient is POD #3 who had a vertical abdominal incision, now with a mass and fever"
What is your differential diagnosis?
How would you evaluate her?

e. "Expanding hematoma in an abdominal incision"
How would you manage? (Candidate packed the wound and obtained an H/H.)
"Her Hb dropped from pre-op of 13 to 7."
What now? The hematoma is still enlarging? (Candidate T&C 2 u PRBC and took her to OR to explore the wound.)
"She has a subcutaneous bleeder which you identify and ligate. How would you close the incision?" (Candidate replied that since it was still POD 0 that he would perform a primary closure.)

2. GI Tract Injuries
    a. Ileus vs. Bowel Obstruction
      i. "You performed a TAH BSO on a patient and she calls with abdominal pain."
What is your differential diagnosis?
How do you evaluate her?
Ileus vs. small bowel obstruction—how do you diagnose?
How do you manage?
What do you see on an abdominal series in ileus vs. obstruction?
How do you manage each?
Okay, it turns out she has an obstruction. What is general surgery going to do?

      ii. "Post-op patient with nausea/vomiting on POD #2, then POD #7 getting progressively worse."
What is your differential diagnosis?
How would you manage?
Compare and contrast the causes and management from POD #2 and POD #7.
Compare the presentation, imaging studies, and management for ileus vs. SBO.
Can you see free air on CT scan? X-ray?

(Candidate's patient had free air on x-ray) What do you do?
(Then the patient had free fluid in the peritoneum)
What is the differential diagnosis? (I went on with intraperitoneal vs. retroperitoneal hematoma, hemorrhage, urinoma, etc.)
(I can't remember anymore. Some folks went on to discuss post-op evaluation of bladder or ureteral injury.)

b. Enterotomy

    i. "You are performing a posterior repair as part of a VH, when you inadvertently make an enterotomy."
Discuss management, repair, surgical technique, post-op care.

    ii. "After a TAH, BSO for a tubo-ovarian abscess, the patient has nausea and vomiting."
Discuss differential diagnosis, work-up, IVF selection, management.
"After 6 days of conservative management, she is no better."
Discuss evaluation.
"A CT shows an 8cm fluid collection in the pelvis."
How do you proceed?
"A KUB shows air/fluid levels and bowel wall edema."
What do you do? How do you repair a bowel injury?

*Case List*
1. S/P TAH, BSO POD #3 with abdominal distension
How do you separate an ileus from an obstruction?
2. S/P laparoscopic BSO, 4 hours post-op with N/V
What is your differential diagnosis?
How do you separate if the cause is a perforation vs. electrocautery injury?
3. How do you repair a serosal tear?
How do you repair a mucosal tear?
How do you repair a transaction of the bowel?

3. Nerve Injuries

    a. "Patient comes in complaining of abdominal pain after a laparotomy located to the anterior abdominal wall."
What is your differential diagnosis?
How would you evaluate each?
"Now they tell you it's a suture entrapment."
What is the nerve that is entrapped how do you manage?
"Now a patient that had a vaginal hysterectomy has foot drop."
What nerve was damaged?
What do you do?
How do you manage her?
What do you tell the patient?
"Now a patient is POD day one and can't walk because her leg buckles."
What nerve was injured?
How did the injury occur?
What can you do to prevent it?
What are other causes of dizziness and being unable to walk post-op day one that are not lower leg related?

    b. Five or six questions all on femoral nerve, lateral peroneal nerve
(This was my first question in GYN, and I was traumatized!!!)
"Post-op patient with difficulties walking"
What is the nerve involved? Femoral nerve or sciatic nerve? (I said femoral.)

How did the injury occur? (self-retaining retractors/hyperflexion of hips in dorsal lithotomy position)
What is the management? (patient reassurance, physical therapy)
How do you counsel the patient? (patient reassurance, physical therapy)
How long before you become concerned? (2-3 months. If symptoms persist, refer to Neurology)
(And there were more and more cases, such as patient with foot drop (peroneal nerve)....Same questions.)

    c. "A 30-year-old, 110-pound patient POD #1 TAH falls secondary to her leg buckling as she attempts to get out of bed."
Discuss your exam. Which nerve is injured? Treatment, prevention.

4. Urological Injuries
    a. * Ureteral injury

        i. "A patient with a broad ligament fibroid is undergoing a TAH. During the surgery, you suspect you may have injured the ureter."

        ii. "Patient in recovery room after a difficult hysterectomy for fibroids, with anuria"
Pre- and intraoperative prevention, recognition, management, three most common sites of ureteral injury.

        iii. "A patient, on whom you did a difficult hysterectomy, presents on POD #2 c/o unilateral back pain."
Discuss differential diagnosis, work-up, presentation if ureteral injury, management.

        iv. "A woman who just had a cesarean delivery passes only 30ml of urine in several hours."
What is your differential diagnosis?
How do you evaluate and treat? (They went down the road of ureteric damage with this one.)

    b. Fistula
        i. Vesicovaginal fistula—"Patient presents 7 days after TVH with continuous vaginal discharge."
What is your differential diagnosis?
How would you evaluate her?
"It is a vesicovaginal fistula."
How would you differentiate between a vesicovaginal fistula and a ureterovaginal? What would be your approach to repair a vesicovaginal fistula? (I tried to pawn it off on Urogyn at almost every step, but they came back with, "Well, say you were to do it yourself.")
"Post-hysterectomy GU fistula"
What is a fistulagram? Presentation, work-up, management
"Postoperative patient, S/P TVH with profuse watery vaginal discharge."
Patient found to have a ureterovaginal fistula.

        ii. Rectovaginal fistula—"Young nulliparous patient presents with a rectovaginal fistula." Discuss differential diagnosis (inflammatory bowel disease), management, colostomy (Y/N).
"A patient S/P SVD 6 weeks ago presents with passing gas/stool from vagina"
What is your differential diagnosis? How would you evaluate her?
"On exam you identify a fistulous tract between the rectum and vagina."
How would you manage her? If you are going to repair her, how long will you wait?

c. Bladder injury
   i. "Patient with a wound draining yellow fluid"
      How do check to see if it's urine? Okay, you sent it off and the creatinine is 18. It's urine. What do you do?
      The urologist is out of town. How do you locate the injury? (imaging, etc.)
      How do you fix the damage etc
      Differential diagnosis of wound drainage
      How do you evaluate it?

   ii. "Patient undergoing abdominal surgery is noted to have frank blood in Foley catheter."
      How do you evaluate the hematuria?

   iii. "Post-op the patient has a significant drop in the Hb."
      What is your differential diagnosis?
      How do you work her up?
      "Imaging reveals a fluid collection in the pelvis."
      How do you manage her now?
      "She has a persistent fluid collection in spite of transfusion."
      What is your differential diagnosis?
      How do you work her up?
      "Ends up with a urinoma."
      When do you resume her anti-coagulation post-op, and how?

d. Neurogenic bladder— "Question on neurogenic bladder, PVR
   What are the causes?
   How would you work it up?
   What pharmacologic options are available? (Candidate chose Bethanechol.)

*Case List*

GU injury

1. Ureteral injury during abdominal hysterectomy. Now I would diagnose it? I said cystoscopy, so then she took me through what you do if you don't see ureteral jets. I said pass stents; she said stents won't pass. I said go from above, dissect into the area to try to identify type of injury. She asked me where/how I would do the dissection. I discussed going into the retroperitoneal space, that I would identify ureter at the pelvic brim and follow it down. She then said it was transected. I asked her how close to bladder. She said near uterine artery, so I said I would then repair with ureteroneocystotomy. She stopped the question at that point.
2. Cystotomy on case list—how did it happen? How can you avoid it in the future?
3. Cystotomy on case list—where was the site of injury? How/when did you recognize it? How long did you drain her? How did you know when to take the catheter out?
4. What is the course of the ureter?

5. Hysterectomy Complications
   a. "A patient is 6 weeks post-op from a TVH, presents with pain, vaginal discharge, and bleeding."
      What is your differential diagnosis?
      How would you evaluate her?
      How would you manage granulation tissue at the vaginal cuff?
      How would you manage fallopian tube prolapse?

b. Bowel prolapse through the cuff

    i. "Patient who is one week S/P TVH presents with open vaginal cuff and loop of small bowel prolapsing through the vaginal cuff. Not necrotic.
How would you manage?

    ii. "Post-operative patient, S/P TVH presents with vaginal fullness. Exam reveals loop of small bowel in the vagina."

    iii. "One year after a VH, a patient presents c/o dyspareunia. On exam, you note a beefy red mass protruding through the cuff."
Symptoms, recognition, management (expectant vs. surgical).

c. "A patient in the recovery room with brisk vaginal bleeding post VH"
How would you evaluate her? (Candidate responded to go back to the OR. The examiner asked, "Why not examine her in PAR?" The candidate replied that if he lifted up the sheet and the bleeding was truly brisk, that he needs to examine her back in the OR under general anesthesia.)
"Okay, there is obvious bleeding from the cuff corner. How would you manage her?"
(Candidate replied that he would place a suture, then perform cystoscopy to assess the ureter. For those who did not perform cystoscopy, the patient ended up with post-op fever and flank pain and ended up with a ligated ureter.)

d. "Patient seen in the office for post-op check for a VH and fimbria are seen prolapsing from the cuff."
How would you manage her? (Candidate replied to treat with AgNO3.)
"She has severe pain. What would you do now?" (Candidate elected to take her to the OR.)
"Would you pull down on the tube?" (Candidate replied absolutely not, that he would place a loop ligature.)
"Let's say you pulled on the tube and you encounter hemorrhage? What would you do?" (Candidate reminded the examiner that he wouldn't have pulled on it in the first place, but now he would have to open the patient with a laparotomy to investigate.)

*Case List*

1. How you counsel someone for route of hysterectomy; abdominal, vaginal, laparoscopic, supracervical?
2. (*Although not a case of the day, coincidentally, everyone on this day had the same line of questioning that stemmed from the case list with a hysterectomy.*)
3. Draw a McCalls culdoplasty. How do you perform a cystoscopy? What do you do if there is no efflux?
4. Define medical management before resorting to a hysterectomy.
5. Why don't you perform more vaginal hysterectomies? How do you determine if a patient is a candidate?
6. From a supracervical hysterectomy
    Why was it done?
    Are there specific scenarios that a supracervical hysterectomy is indicated?
    What are the landmarks that you look for when doing a supracervical hysterectomy?
    What do you do if the patient returns to clinic POD #7 with vaginal bleeding? How do you counsel?
    What do you do if the patient returns to clinic POD #7 with copious watery discharge? How do you counsel?
    How do you counsel her about Pap tests?
    What if she continued to have cyclic bleeding? How do you counsel?

7. Supracervical hysterectomy
How do you counsel the patient?
If your pathology comes back with uterine cancer, what do you do with the cervix?
8. From a TVH
"Take us through the steps that you do in performing a VH."
What if you were trying to get in anteriorly and a large gush of fluid came out?"
How would you repair a cystotomy during a VH?
How do you support your vaginal cuff in a VH?
9. From a VH—How do you support the cuff? Describe your specific method step by step.
10. Discussed decision to perform LAVH vs. TVH. When to do laparoscopy.
11. Discussed differential diagnosis for 44-year-old female with persistent multiloculated 5cm ovarian masses. Discussed when to do a BSO. How do you counsel a patient for a BSO?
12. They asked a lot about alternatives to hysterectomy (e.g., new *Compendium* article) (These questions were reasonable. I can't remember anything that was too hard…mostly what I tried before surgery.)
13. I had a lot of TLH, LAVH, LSH on the case list. Where is the inferior epigastric artery? How do you identify it in a patient with BMI of 50? How do you remove the uterus? The candidate responded with the morcellator. The examiner then asked what happens if you accidentally step on the pedal and the morcellator barrels into the patient? The candidate replied that his morcellator trigger is hand held, but nonetheless given the severity of injury, opened the patient up to investigate the severity of damage.

6. Fibroids

   *Case List*

   1. Myomectomy—What is the role of uterine artery embolization?

   2. Used a D&C hysteroscopy case to ask about alternative managements for fibroids. Asked about the patient I had specifically (submucosal fibroid) and in a general sense.
   They were only looking for types of management, not how you actually do any of the management.
   E.g., Lupron, UAE, resection with hysteroscopy, ablation, myomectomy hysterectomy.

   3. How does uterine leiomyoma cause uterine bleeding?

   4. How I would make an incision on a patient with a large fibroid uterus, whose prior vertical skin incision moved with the uterus during the bimanual exam?

7. * Laparoscopic complications:

   "You note a large volume of blood dripping down the sleeve after passage of the LLQ trochar" or "You note an expanding retroperitoneal hematoma when you pass the camera for a LTL."
   What vessel did you injure?
   Discuss the anatomy of the inferior epigastric artery, management, prevention.

Laparoscopy

   *Case List*
   Used a generic laparoscopic case.
   How do I do a laparoscopy? (I had to ask for clarification.
   They were interested in entry vs. needle vs. open vs. direct.)
   Where do I put my ports?
   What am I or should I be worried about with placing trocars?

What landmarks do I use to place my trocars?
What is the anatomy of the inferior epigastric vessels?
Do the inferior epigastric vessels go above or below the fascia?

## D. Urogynecology

1. *Prolapse

   a. "A 75-year-old who underwent VH with A and P repair presents with total vaginal vault eversion with ulcerations."
      Discuss steps for prevention, evaluation, treatment.

   b. "A 75-year-old presents with procidentia."
      Where do you make the initial incision for a VH? Discuss pre-op evaluation, recommendations for surgery, prevention post-op UI or ureteral injury.

   c. "Patient with vaginal vault prolapse"
      What is your technique to support the cuff for Grade 1?
      What is your technique to support the cuff for Grade 3?

   d. "A patient S/P rectovaginal repair, now with rectal pain"
      What is your differential diagnosis?
      How would you work her up?
      How would you treat her?

   e. "Enterocele"
      How do you examine the patient for it? What are you looking for ?
      How do you counsel the patient on the surgical procedure to be performed? how do you explain it to her?
      What is the urogynecologist going to do in the OR?

   f. "Prolapse"
      Enterocele, rectocele, cystocele
      How to evaluate for each
      What are the abdominal repair vs. vaginal repair options?
      How do you perform a sacrospinous ligament fixation?

   g. "Patient is S/P TAHBSO, later had a cystocele repair and now has a vaginal bulge"
      What is your differential diagnosis? (I said prolapsed bowel, vaginal neoplasia, failed anterior repair with recurrent cystocele, apical defect, and posterior wall defect. Then the examiner asked me the other name for apical defect. I said vaginal vault prolapse.)
      How you do evaluate?
      Patient found to have an enterocele. How you manage?
      By this time that word threw me into panic. Why? I don't know, so I said something awful.
      They wanted you do to a vaginal vault suspension, depending if you said abdominal sacrocoplexy or sacrospinous ligament fixation. They asked you to explain why you chose either route, to describe the procedure, and to indicate what vessels/nerves that you would injure.

   h. "You are performing a TOT and encounter brisk bleeding at the skin when you deliver the trochar."
      How would you manage the patient? (Candidate responded pressure.)
      "After 10 minutes of pressure, the bleeding is worse, what now?" (Candidate wanted to call in interventional radiology if she were stable. Of course, he was unavailable.) What now? Candidate took her back to the OR to open the space of Retzius to explore the obturator artery.

*Case List*

## Pelvic organ prolapse (POP)

Define the stages/grades
Abdominal sacral colposuspension
How would you counsel a patient? (no questions on technique)
Sacrospinous ligament fixation (SSLF)
What are the spaces that you course to gain access to the SSL?
What do you do if you encounter bleeding after you place your suture in the SSL?
How do you counsel a patient with POP? How do your treatment options change if she does not have concurrent incontinence? How do you evaluate UI pre-op?
What type of pessaries do you use? Why? How do you instruct the patient on self-care? How do you instruct a patient who wants you to manage her pessary?
How can you prevent apical vaginal vault prolapse?

2. *Urinary Incontinence
   a. "A 56-year-old present with c/o urinary incontinence with coughing and sneezing." Describe the work-up (standing stress test, Q-tip), differentiation from overactive bladder, surgical and conservative management.

   b. TVT/TOT Complications—"Patient had a TVT and now has urinary retention."
   How do you manage her?
   How do you evaluate her?
   "So you tried a Foley and that doesn't fix her retention."
   Now what do you do?
   "So you teach her clean intermittent self catheterization."
   For how long?
   "Okay, now she's fed up and doesn't want to do that anymore."
   Basically they push you into taking her back to the OR to cut the tape.
   What do you tell her in terms of her continence?
   What percent of patients are still continent ever after you cut the tape?
   "Now another patient had a TVT and comes in with frequency urgency and hematuria." Basically, she has an erosion of the tape.
   How do you diagnose and manage?
   I had a bladder erosion that the urologist came and took out and fixed the bladder in layers; another candidate had a vaginal erosion that she cut out and re-approximated and then gave the lady vaginal Premarin cream.

*Case List*

1. How do you work up urinary incontinence in the office?
2. TVH combined case with urogyn TVT
Asked about retention.
How do you manage urinary retention after TVT?
Retention after 2 days?
Retention after 1 week?
Retention after 2 weeks?
How was this patient diagnosed with GSUI?
Did she need urodynamics?

3. Interstitial cystitis
How do you diagnose interstitial cystitis? If you perform hydrodistention but she still has symptoms, how do you treat her now? What other diagnostic tests are available? How accurate are they?

## E. Infections

1. PID

   a. "You are consulted intraoperatively by a general surgeon for a 19-year-old with PID. You identify a pyosalpinx and ovarian adhesions."
   Discuss medical and surgical options, antibiotic selection, preservation of fertility, criteria for inpatient management.

   b. "A patient is hospitalized for PID."
   Discuss antibiotic selection.
   "The patient is noted to be hypotensive and tachycardic."
   Discuss differential diagnosis (answer: septic shock); management (including Swan-Ganz catheter). Taken to OR. What type of surgery? Noted to have bilateral tubo-ovarian abscess. What would you do? Unable to perform TAH, BSO 2° adhesions—supracervical hysterectomy, BSO. How do you counsel the patient afterwards? Would you start HRT? If so, which one?

2.* Post-op fever

   a. "A patient is noted to have a temperature of 101.5° F. on POD #3."
   Discuss differential diagnosis, work-up, and management, especially if fever unresponsive to antibiotics, antibiotic selection.

   b. POD #2 S/P TVH patient has T102 and 4 cm mass at cuff"
   Evaluation
   Diagnosis
   Management

   Other questions: Here they really pushed about what antibiotics, when or if you would do a CT and when or if you would take her back to the OR. If you took her back to the OR, how would you drain or treat, specifically in the OR?

   There was a case on endometritis that just wasn't getting better on antibiotics and ending up having septic pelvic thrombophlebitis and you had to start Heparin.

   There was a case of endometritis that was on prolonged antibiotics and kept spiking and ended up having diarrhea *C. diff*. What do you do? Do you stop antibiotics? How do you check for *C. diff*? How do you treat? What are all of the treatment options?

## F. Abnormal Bleeding

1. "A 36-year-old presents with menorrhagia and is found to have an endometrial polyp on hysteroscopy."
   Discuss diagnosis, management.

2. Imperforate hymen—"A virginal female c/o vaginal blockage when first attempting intercourse"
   Discuss diagnosis, embryology management—surgical vs. non-surgical (dilators).

3. PMPB

   a. "A 64-year-old has vaginal spotting x3 weeks and is not on HRT."
   Discuss differential diagnosis, work-up, management.

   b. "An 89-year-old demented patient from the nursing home has vaginal bleeding."

   c. "64-year-old female with 3-month history of brown vaginal discharge"
   What is your differential diagnosis?
   How would you evaluate her?
   What if she had lower back pain?
   Discuss differential diagnosis, work-up, management.

    d. "A 70-year-old woman with a brown vaginal discharge"
How do you evaluate her?
"You perform an endometrial biopsy which shows atypical hyperplasia."
How do you counsel her?

4. "A 21-year-old had rough intercourse and is noted to have brisk vaginal bleeding and a laceration in the posterior cul-de-sac."
Discuss evaluation, management (laparoscopy vs. laparotomy).

5. Anemia

    a. "A patient with anemia preoperatively"
Definition of anemia, work-up, management, timing for surgery.

    b. "A patient in her 20s-30s with post-op anemia. Hb = 18"
When would you transfuse her?
What is your transfusion goal?
What are the risks associated with transfusion?

    c. "You get called by a nurse to say that your patient was accidentally transfused with the wrong patient's blood."
What do you tell her to do?
What are major transfusion reactions?
What are minor reactions?
How do you manage them?

6. Cervical polyp –"A 39-year-old with fleshy, polypoid cervical mass"
Discuss differential diagnosis, management of asymptomatic vs. bleeding patient.

7. "A 35-year-old with 14-week size uterus with vaginal bleeding and menorrhagia, causing her to miss two weeks of work in the last few months."
What is your differential diagnosis?
How do you evaluate her?
What labs would you order?
How would you manage her?

8. Hysteroscopy

    a. "A patient had a D&C one week ago and presents with fever and abdominal pain."
What is your differential diagnosis?
How do you evaluate her?
How do you manage her?

    b. "You are planning a D&C and have difficulty dilating the cervix. You note a sudden loss of resistance and note profuse bleeding."
How do you assess for a uterine perforation?
Describe the anatomy of the uterine artery and how you would achieve hemostasis if the vessel was injured.

    c. "Patient is S/P endometrial ablation with fever, chills, and acute abdominal pain."
What is your differential diagnosis? (Candidate responded: Septic AB, PID, TOA, ovarian torsion, appendicitis, pancreatitis, cholecystitis)
How do you evaluate and manage? (VS, O2 sat, abdominal exam, pelvic exam, cultures, pelvic U/S, blood cultures, urine cultures, CBC. Admit, IV broad spectrum antibiotics.)
I think the patient had endometritis. How long will you continue IV antibiotics?
What bacteria are involved? What do you use as outpatient?

    d. "A patient that wanted to have an endometrial ablation with a 12-week uterus"
How do you counsel her on options, risks, and benefits? (I discussed complications such as uterine perforation, thermal injury, electrolyte imbalances....Nope!!

They pushed and asked, "What else?" So I finally started babbling about contraception and pregnancy complications. And they listened.)
He wanted all of the info regarding ablations: how do you counsel her on percentage of failure rates, amenorrhea rates, etc.
Then you are asked about Uterine Artery Embolization (UAE)
Options, risks, and benefits
Failure rates
Complications. (I started discussing perforation of uterine artery, bowel....babbling. Then the examiner stated the patient now has hot flushes. I then stated, "Possible embolization of ovarian artery or collaterals leading to decreased ovarian function and menopause," and the examiner moved on.
"What if a she has UAE and now comes back pregnant?"
How do you counsel and now manage the pregnancy?

*Case List*

1. Distension medium, why you wouldn't use electrolyte medium with cautery, fluid deficits for isotonic and hypotonic medium, when to stop the procedure, how would you monitor the patient post-op, what labs would you order, would you admit her
2. Perforation—management depending upon location
3. What distension fluid do you use? How do you monitor for volume overload? If you perforate the uterus, when do you perform a laparoscopy? Would your management change if you suspect a lateral vascular injury? If you perform a laparotomy, what are you looking for?
4. Why did you do a D&C hysteroscopy on a 25-, 26-, 27, 28-, and 29- year-old? Did they all refuse an office endometrial biopsy? Do you have access to saline sonohystograms?
5. Why do you do a D&C hysteroscopy with your ablations? What if it comes back endometrial hyperplasia? Lots of questions on management of hyperplasia with and without atypia, both simple and complex
6. How to evaluate and treat menometrorrhagia before hysterectomy
7. Uterine artery embolization—side effects, benefits, reproductive capacity afterwards.

## G. Perioperative Management

1. Preoperative/perioperative evaluation
    a. "Preoperative/perioperative evaluation and management"
    A 25-year-old with asthma, well controlled
    A 35-year-old DM scheduled for a BTL.
    Specifically what do you do about meds for Type I or Type II on orals? What would you do if the case was bumped?
    A 40-year-old healthy female scheduled for a hysterectomy
    Other questions:
    What are my pre-op antibiotics?
    Are there situations where I would redose the antibiotic?

    b. "You are seeing a morbidly obese patient pre-op for a hysterectomy."
    How do you counsel the patient?
    What measures do you take to prevent DVT?
    What measures to you take to prevent pneumonia?

    c. "You are seeing a patient pre-op for a hysterectomy who has a history of DVT and PE."
    How do you manage her Coumadin? (Candidate bridged from Coumadin to Heparin.)
    How do you instruct her on her Heparin immediate pre-op?

When do you resume Heparin post-op?

"2 days post-op she has a massive PE."

How do you manage her? (Candidate responded ABCs and Heparin.)

What loading dose of Heparin? (Candidate responded he would consult the intensivist or hospitalist, but examiner replied they were unavailable.)

How do you put her back on the Coumadin? When can she go home?

d. "A 60-year-old on Plavix for acute coronary syndrome needs hysterectomy."

How do you manage the Plavix preoperatively?

"A 48-year-old with a mechanical heart valve on Coumadin"

How do you manage the Coumadin preoperatively for a scheduled case?

How do you manage the Coumadin preoperatively for an emergent case?

How do you manage the Coumadin postoperatively?

e. "A patient with a history of DVT 3 years ago after child was born. Negative w/u."

How do you handle her peri-op? (scheduled for TAH)

They asked lots of questions about how long/doses/Heparin vs. Lovenox/risks of the meds, including HITS

f. A patient with anti-phospholipid Ab with history of arterial thrombosis"

Discuss perioperative management, Coumadin vs. Lovenox, when to restart, how to reverse.

g. Hypokalemia—"A patient's pre-op labs reveal a potassium of 2.3."

Discuss differential diagnosis, symptoms, risks, management.

h. HIV—"A 30-year-old HIV+ patient is scheduled for an indicated hysterectomy."

Perioperative precautions (for patient—How would you manage? Any tests?

Intraoperative precautions

"In the surgery, the scrub tech gets a needle stick."

What do you do?

What evaluation does the patient with the needle stick injury get?

What treatment are they given and for how long?

i. "A diabetic patient is noted to have a blood sugar of 200 the morning of surgery."

Discuss management.

j. "A patient with a history of several previous abdominal surgeries comes in for a pre-op evaluation. The abdominal wall moves upon manipulation of the cervix."

What do you do?

How do you proceed with surgery

k. Discuss your work-up for a 40-year-old scheduled for a TAH.

When would you consider a CXR and an EKG?

2. Chest pain

"An 81-year-old who underwent TAH and BSO for endometrial cancer with shortness of breath and chest pain"

Discuss work-up, differential diagnosis, V/Q scan interpretation and influence on management. How do you diagnose an acute myocardial infarction (AMI) on EKG? What laboratory tests should you order for AMI? Could her presentation be simply atelectasis?

3. Shortness of Breath

a. "A female POD #2 from a hysterectomy with shortness of breath and tachycardia"

What is your differential diagnosis?

How would you work her up?

"Patient has a PE." How would you manage her?

b. PE:

Discuss differential diagnosis, work-up, V/Q scans (sensitivity/specificity), treatment, Heparin vs. LMWH (mechanism of action, dose, complications, monitoring), prevention.

4. Shock

a. "A 65-year-old who has just undergone a TAH, BSO for endometrial cancer. In the recovery room, she develops hypotension, tachycardia, tachypnea, and decreased urine output."

Discuss differential diagnosis, treatment, pulmonary embolus, shock.

b. "A patient presents two weeks after having a VH. She had intercourse a few hours earlier and now presents with severe lower abdominal pain, vaginal bleeding, tachycardia, hypotension."

Describe work-up, management, blood replacement therapy.

5. Hypoxia

"You are called on a patient who is POD #1 from a TAH, a former heroin addict, with an O2 saturation of 90%, respiratory rate of 10, and difficult to arouse."

What is your differential diagnosis?

How would you manage her?

"She is now POD #3 and has mental status changes, delirium, and agitation."

How would you evaluate her?

How would you manage her?

## H. Sterilization

1. "You perform a modified Pomeroy PPTL."

How do you counsel the patient re: immediate vs. delayed sterilization? Justify your method of choice.

"The histology report shows full thickness of tube on only one side."

How do you counsel the patient? How do you evaluate her?

"At the end of the procedure you see blood rising in the field."

What would you do?

"At laparotomy, you see a broad ligament hematoma."

What would you do?

2. "A 34-year-old desires sterilization."

Options/counseling regarding failure rates

"You perform a laparoscopic Filshie clip and get 3cm hematoma in broad ligament."

What are your management options?

*Case List*

Failure rates of a laparoscopic tubal ligation, Essure

Counseling patient on sterilization options

## I. Endometriosis

1. "A 21-year-old with chronic pelvic pain undergoes a laparoscopy and is noted to have endometrial implants on both ovaries and the pelvic sidewalls and cul-de-sac."

Discuss surgical options, counseling re: TAH and/or BSO, medical options (including GNRH and add-back therapy).

2. "4 days after TAH and BSO for severe endometriosis, a 31-year-old complains of severe hot flushes."

Discuss role of HRT, risks of reactivating residual endometriosis, alternative to HRT.

*Case List*
1. What are the treatment options?
2. GnRH agonists, OCPs?
What is the mechanism of action?
How do you prescribe them?
How do you instruct your patients on their use?
What are side effects?
3. What are the expected surgical findings?

## I. Other

1. Leiomyomata—"A 35-year-old 3G/0P c/o chronic lower abdominal pain attributed to an enlarged multifibroid uterus. She also has a history of three prior second trimester pregnancy losses."
   Discuss evaluation, management—open vs. laparoscopic vs. hysteroscopic myomectomy.

2. Dysmenorrhea—"26-year-old 0G with severe dysmenorrhea misses two days of work monthly, has no relief with NSAIDs, and has negative diagnostic laparoscopy."
   Etiologies? Next step?

---

# TABLE 3   Office Practice

---

## A. *Preventative Care and Health Maintenance

1. Osteoporosis
   a. "Postmenopausal patient with history of breast carcinoma in situ two years ago develops osteoporosis."
   Discuss counseling about HRT, other options, T vs. Z score.

   b. "A 67-year-old female with T score of -2.5 and smoker"
   What is her diagnosis, and how would you screen?
   What are her and in general risk factors?
   How do you treat? (The examiners really beat me up on all the types and options. Thankfully, I was prepared )

2. *Well woman/Immunizations
   a. "A 19-year-old virgin, college-bound, comes for a routine annual exam."
   What vaccinations would you recommend?
   What is the Gardasil vaccine?
   What percent of dysplasia/genital warts does it protect against?
   "The patient's mom wants to know when her first Pap smear should be. What do you advise?"
   "The patient desires contraception."
   What are her options if she has irregular bleeding?
   What are her options if she has menorrhagia?
   "Her menses have always been heavy ,resulting in anemia."
   What is your differential diagnosis?
   How would you work up von Willebrands disease?

b. "A 60-year-old with unremarkable past medical history"
   What is routine screening?
   What immunizations would you recommend?

Case List
1. Which vaccinations are recommended for various age groups?
2. Annual health exam: created multiple permutations with different ages of patients on what screening tests and vaccines should be offered. Asked when I would initiate lipid, thyroid screening, diabetes screening, focused a lot on bone density screening and the details of that. They asked me if the treatments differed between a patient with osteopenia and osteoporosis
3. When would you order a DEXA scan?
4. What do you recommend for routine screening depending on age group?
5. What vaccinations would you recommend in a 21-year-old?
6. How do you counsel a 78-year-old re: preventative care? Do you recommend Pap smears?
7. When to start screening for mammograms, thyroid disease, diabetes, cholesterol, bone density. Discussed risk factors and treatment of osteoporosis. What if her T score was 1.4? What if it was 2?
8. Discussed what immunizations to give for a 53-year-old woman.

## B. * Counseling for Smoking Cessation and Treatment of Obesity

1. "A 65-year-old who smokes two packs of cigarettes daily is 30% overweight and has not seen a doctor for 30 years."
   What aspects of the exam do you emphasize? How do you calculate the BMI? How do you counsel for weight loss (diet, exercise, medications)? How do you counsel for smoking cessation (stop date, gum, patch, medications).

   *Case List*
   Patient with obesity
   How do you calculate the BMI?
   What is the definition of obesity?

## C. Sexual Dysfunction

1. Dyspareunia
   a. "Patient who underwent SVD 7 months ago complains of introital dyspareunia."
      Discuss differential diagnosis, treatment.

   b. "A 27-year-old is 7 months post partum and c/o entry dyspareunia."
      Discuss differential diagnosis, evaluation, and management.

   c. "A patient is two months post-op from a TVH, posterior colporrhaphy. She complains of pain, dyspareunia, and vaginal discharge"
      What is your differential diagnosis?
      "You feel a firm mass below the site of the posterior repair."
      What is your differential diagnosis? How would you evaluate her?

2. Libido—"A patient c/o decreased libido."
   Discuss differential diagnosis, counseling, treatment.

   *Case List*
   1. Sexual dysfunction and body image –how do I counsel? (I believe I was asked why would I refer my obese patient with body image issues and low libido to couples therapy. I justified that referral by focusing on relationship dynamics, stressors such as job loss, finances....babbling....)

## D. *Contraception

1. IUD

   a. "A 29-year-old insulin-dependent diabetic wants an IUD."
      Discuss counseling, contraindications, risks (including ectopic pregnancy),
      management of abnormal bleeding (differential diagnosis including pregnancy,
      management if she became pregnant—counseling, removal).

   b. "A patient in the first trimester is pregnant with an IUD in situ."
      How would you manage her?

   c. "A 23-year-old female follow up from Mirena IUD and no strings are visible"
      How do you evaluate her?
      "A sonogram does not show the IUD."
      What do you do next?
      "A sonogram shows the IUD."
      How do you remove it?
      What if the IUD is perforated? How do you work her up? How do you remove it?
      "Now she comes in 8 weeks pregnant, and you can see the strings."
      What do you do?
      How do you counsel the patient?
      What do you do if you can't see the string?

   d. "Patient had IUD placed postpartum and comes in with fever, abdominal pain
      and purulent discharge."
      How do you remove the IUD?
      "Now her fever is 102.4° F. and she's basically getting septic."
      How do you manage ?
      "So now she's in the hospital and still spiking and not getting better.
      She eventually develops an abscess, and you have to manage it."
      When do you just drain it? When do you do a TAH BSO?

   e. "Patient with an IUD and missing strings"
      How do you evaluate? (I immediately asked for LMP and HCG test, which
      determines my management.)
      "Negative HCG. What do you do?"
      Speculum exam, use cytobrush to sweep strings, if unsuccessful, obtain pelvic
      U/S to determine location of IUD. If displaced, remove via hysteroscopy. If in
      normal position, leave in situ or offer removal/replacement. "Positive HCG."
      Do U/S to determine if IUP vs. ectopic. If IUP and first trimester, counsel patient
      on risk of PTB and SAB and recommend removal. Use cytobrush to sweep
      strings. The examiner stated strings still unobtainable. Then I asked if patient
      desired this pregnancy; if so, then I would leave in situ and counsel patient. If
      patient does not desire pregnancy, recommend hysteroscopic removal and EAB.

   f. "Patient with mucopurulent discharge and IUD"
      What is your differential diagnosis?
      How do you evaluate and manage?
      Depending on when cervicitis is diagnosed in relation to time of insertion,
      patient's history, and risk for unintended pregnancy, I kept the IUD in situ. I was
      asked what would be my criteria to remove the IUD?
      "Persistent or worsening sx's. What would be my criteria to admit to hospital?"
      Pregnancy, TOA, unable to tolerate po meds, noncompliance, etc.
      "What antibiotics would I start as an outpatient?"
      Ceftriaxone 250mg IM and Doxycycline 100mg bidiagnosis 14 days
      "What antibiotics would I start as an inpatient?"
      Cefotetan 2gm IV q12h and Doxy 100mg IV q12h

g. "Case of the day on IUD"
   Acute PID with IUD intact
   Pregnancy with IUD
   lost IUD w/u

2. Oral Contraception
   "Patient with lupus requests OCPs."
   "Type I diabetic requests contraception"
   If she has hypertension, what contraceptive option would you offer her?
   What are the advantages and disadvantages of OCPs, IUD and barrier techniques?
   What if the patient had SLE?

3. Emergency Contraception
   A 22-year-old nulliparous wants emergency contraception"
   Criteria for EC
   Options
   Success/failure rates of each

4. General Counseling
   How do you counsel for and what is the failure for …?
   Essure vs. IUD vs. BTL
   Multiple questions regarding IUD insertion/side effects, contraceptive patch, Essure

   Case List

   Contraception
   1. Emergency contraception: options, efficacy, side effects
   2. Contraindications of OCPs particularly in a patient with prior DVT.
   3. The patient conceives with an IUD in place. How would you manage her? If the U/S shows an 8-week viable IUP, how would you proceed? If the U/S shows a 20-week IUP, how would you proceed?
   4. How do you decide which IUD to use?
   5. What are contraindications to OCPS?
   6. Discussed indications/contraindications for placement of IUD, the two available options, risks/benefits of each. What would you do if the IUD was not visible at her 4-week checkup? What if the ultrasound didn't show the IUD? What would you do if the abdominal x-ray showed an intraperitoneal IUD? What if the Pap smear showed actinomycosis?

## E. Genetic and Preconception Counseling

1. "Your OG patient has a sister with a Factor 5 Leiden mutation."
   How would you work her up, counsel, and manage her pregnancy?

2. "25-year-old with IDDM desires conception."
   How do you counsel her re: risks to her and the baby?

   "Her HbA1C = 10. What serum glucose does that correlate with and how does that influence your counseling?" (We all agree that's not good, but no one knew what it correlated with. We checked with an internist, who stated there are charts for reference and that it would = an average glucose of 300-320.)

## F. *Amenorrhea

1. "A 15-year-old with primary amenorrhea"
   Discuss etiologies (primary vs. secondary amenorrhea), work-up (reveals blind vaginal pouch), diagnosis (reveals testicular feminization).

2. "A 52-year-old who has been amenorrheic for one year presents for annual exam." Discuss evaluation, routine screens, laboratory test, HRT counseling.

3. "Asherman's Syndrome"
   Discuss who is at risk, treatment (hysteroscopic resection—distension media, detection and treatment of water intoxication, post-op management).

4. "An athlete marathon runner presents with amenorrhea." What is she at risk for? How would you treat her?

## G.*PCOS, Hirsutism

1. "A 20-year-old c/o hirsutism and oligomenorrhea. Her mom and sister had similar complaints."
   Discuss differential diagnosis, work-up, laboratory tests, presentation, management, medications (types, mechanism of action).

2. "An infertile, hirsute, obese female with oligomenorrhea"
   How do you evaluate her?
   What are the long term risks of PCOS?
   How do you screen for them? (DM, HTN, dyslipidemia)
   How do you treat her?

3. "An 18-year-old, obese, oligomenorrhea, with hirsutism"
   What is your differential diagnosis?
   Evaluation
   Diagnostic criteria for PCOS

4. "A 37-year-old with new onset hirsutism" and "a 19-year-old with hirsutism and acne"
   What labs would you order?
   How would you treat them?

5. "A 26-year-old gains 60 pounds within 6 months."
   What is your differential diagnosis and how will you evaluate her?
   What is the metabolic syndrome?
   How do you treat?

## H. Infertility

1. "A 26-year-old taking OCPs for the past 10 years has a history of oligomenorrhea and was placed on OCPs as a teenager; she now desires pregnancy."
   Discuss counseling.

2. "A27-year-old 1G/0P/el Ab1 with a one-year history of infertility with a partner who fathered two children in a previous marriage."
   Discuss work-up, causes of unexplained infertility, treatment of anovulvatory infertility.

3. "An infertile couple, with marital discord, with premature ejaculation."
   Would you examine him?

4. "A 38-year-old 0G with irregular menses and three years of infertility and a normal semen analysis"
   What is your differential diagnosis?
   What laboratory evaluation would you obtain?
   How would you assess for ovulation? "You diagnose anovulation."
   How would you treat the patient? (Candidate wanted to refer to REI, but the examiner states the patient refused the referral.)
   How do you assess for ovarian hyperstimulation?
   How would you treat her ovarian hyperstimulation?

5. "A 25-year-old marathon runner presents with amenorrhea."
   What is your differential diagnosis?
   How would you work her up?
   "She now wants to get pregnant."
   How would you manage her?

6. "Infertility patient with enlarged uterus on exam"
   What is your differential diagnosis?
   How would you work her up?
   "Sonogram reveals leiomyoma."
   Would you obtain any additional imaging? (Candidate responded sonohysterogram)
   How would you counsel her on her options? (hysteroscopic vs. open myomectomy vs. laparoscopic)
   How do you decide if it can be done hysteroscopically?
   "Okay, she has a 5cm, post-fibroid entering the broad ligament."
   What do you recommend? (Candidate responded to open. They pressured me to take it out laparoscopically since there was only one. I said I was not comfortable.)
   What are the risks of myomectomy?
   How do you counsel the patient?

7. "A patient with amenorrhea and infertility"
   How do you evaluate?
   How would you work her up?
   "What if she also has galactorrhea?"
   How would you evaluate her?
   How would you treat her?
   "If the patient is on Bromocriptine, how do you follow her?"
   How do you manage her if she wants to get pregnant?

8. "Recurrent aborter patient"
   How do you work her up?( including labs)
   What is your differential diagnosis?
   How would you treat her if she were APA positive?
   When do you start the Heparin?
   When do you stop?
   How do you counsel her on the risks of pregnancy?

   *Case List*
   Case with Clomid:
   What is secondary infertility? How do you work it up?
   What does the HSG tell you?
   What were the results of the semen analysis?
   How does the Clomid challenge test work?
   How do you know whether or not she ovulated on Clomid?

## I. Endometriosis

"A 20-year-old c/o dysmenorrhea and dyspareunia for one year."
Discuss differential diagnosis, evaluation (endometriosis), management of endometriosis (medical vs. surgical).

*Case List*
1. What other treatment options are available besides GnRH agonists?
2. Case with endometriosis—differential diagnosis, Depo-Lupron—mechanism of action, add back therapy. How long do you keep her on it? At laparoscopy, how do you treat endometriosis that you see?

## J. Hyperprolactinemia

"A 37-year-old presents with a bilateral nipple discharge."
Discuss differential diagnosis, work-up (reveals elevated prolactin), management (Bromocriptine vs. Dostinex—dose, side effects, use in pregnancy).

*Case List*

1. Discussed workup and treatment of hyperprolactinemia, when to start meds, when to stop meds if pregnancy occurred.

## K. Breast Disease

1. <u>Breast mass</u> –
    a. "A 45-year-old with a palpable 3cm breast mass in the LUOQ"
    Discuss work-up (mammogram, ultrasound, FNA) and treatment (given the diagnosis of fibroadenoma, excision).

    b. "A 27-year-old presents with a firm, solid breast lump."
    Discuss work-up (mammogram, ultrasound, FNA) and treatment (given the diagnosis of fibroadenoma, excision).

    c. "A 45-year-old nulliparous patient presents with a 1cm firm, rubbery breast mass. A mammogram three months ago was normal."
    Discuss differential diagnosis, evaluation, management.

    d. "A 20-year-old with a 2cm solid breast mass"
    How would you manage her? (Candidate wanted to wait until after her next menses)
    "The mass persists. What would you do now?" (Candidate ordered an ultrasound)
    "The ultrasound demonstrates a solid mass. What would you do now?"
    (Candidate referred to the GNS and a biopsy showed a fibroadenoma)

    e. "A 40-year-old presents with a cystic mass."
    How would you manage her? (Candidate chose aspiration, which was straw colored.)

    f. "A 56-year-old has a 1cm mass just behind the nipple."
    How would you manage her? (Candidate chose a mammogram.)
    "The mammogram shows a suspicious mass, but cannot rule out a cyst."
    How would you manage her?" (Candidate chose an ultrasound.)
    "The U/S shows a solid mass."
    How would you manage her? (candidate chose to refer for a biopsy)

    g. "A pregnant patient complains of a breast nodule."
    How would you evaluate her?
    "Exam reveals a 4cm mass in the right breast."
    What now? (Candidate ordered U/S.)
    "The ultrasound shows a solid mass."
    What now? (Candidate wanted to refer to GNS, but GNS was unavailable, so recommended biopsy.)
    "Biopsy shows intraductal carcinoma."
    What now? (Candidate recommended lumpectomy.)
    "Patient is 23 weeks EGA now. Would you recommend chemotherapy?"

2. <u>Nipple discharge</u>

    "A 22-year-old 2G/1P with a bilateral white nipple discharge"
    How would you evaluate her?

"A premenopausal female with a green nipple discharge"
What is your differential diagnosis?
How would you evaluate her?
"A 47-year-old with a blood nipple discharge"
How would you evaluate her?

3. Mastitis
   a. "A patient, who is nursing, presents five days post partum with a painful swollen breast with a fever of 100.5° F."
   Discuss differential diagnosis (engorgement vs. mastitis), work-up, management, microbiology, antibiotic selection, when to take to OR.

   b. "A postpartum patient with red breast, temperature 102.4° F.
   What is your differential diagnosis?
   How would you treat her?
   "Would you call in for an antibiotic overnight without exam?
   (They really pressured me to call them in. I refused.)
   "Patient returns a week later with same symptoms"
   How would you treat her now? (I did cultures/breast sonogram to rule out abscess.)
   "Diagnosis: abscess"
   How would you treat her?  When to drain?  How?  Talk through procedure.

   c. "A postpartum patient with temperature of 100.9° F. and bilateral breast tenderness"
   What is your differential diagnosis?
   How would you work her up?

## L *Endocrine Diseases (Diabetes, Thyroid, Adrenal)

1. Diabetes
   a. "Postmenopausal patient with elevated HgA1C."
   Discuss Type I vs. Type II, management. (Do not dwell on who ordered the test in the first place or for what reason)

   b. Discuss your work-up for a young Type I diabetic undergoing a tubal ligation.

2. Thyroid Disease

   a. "A patient has an enlarged thyroid gland. Her TSH is elevated and her free T4 is decreased."
   What is your differential diagnosis?
   How would you evaluate her?
   "An U/S demonstrates a diffusely enlarged gland."
   What is your diagnosis? (Candidate replied Hashimoto's thyroiditis.)
   How would you treat her?

   b. "A patient comes in for annual exam and you palpate an enlarged thyroid gland, but the patient is asymptomatic."
   How do you evaluate her?
   "She is found to have Hashimoto's hypothyroidism."
   How do you manage her?
   What medications do you use?
   When do you recheck TSH?
   What are the long-term effects of untreated hypothyroidism?
   What other autoimmune diseases are associated with hypothyroidism

c. "Reproductive-aged woman with goiter"
How do you evaluate?
You find she has low T3, low T4, and high TSH. How do you treat and manage?
Later, you find she has Hashimoto's thyroiditis. How do you counsel her on
impact of gynecological and obstetrical risk factors?

d. Case of the day on depression—Wanted differential diagnosis. They were looking
for hypothyroidism, which I knew, but missed. They then asked me about how
I would replace thyroid hormone and when to re-evaluate after replacement
started. Thankfully, I knew that one!

## M. Dysmenorrhea

1. "A 15-year-old with primary dysmenorrhea, nausea, vomiting, and headache."
Discuss differential diagnosis, work-up, management.

2. "A young girl with dysmenorrhea and dyspareunia"
What is your differential diagnosis?
How would you work her up?
"Normal exam and sonogram"
How would you treat her? (I said NSAIDS, continuous OCPs)
"She has failed treatment"
Now what? (Basically, we discussed empiric Lupron vs. surgery and when surgery
would be a better option.)

## N. Menopause

1. HRT
   a. "A 60-year-old on cyclic HRT presents with spotting."
   Discuss work-up, treatment.

   b. "A 63-year-old is on the estrogen patch and complains of irregular bleeding. You
   perform an endometrial biopsy, which shows simple hyperplasia without atypia."
   Discuss counseling, treatment.

2. "A 47-year-old S/P TAH, BSO for a well differentiated adenocarcinoma of the uterus now
with dyspareunia and climacteric symptoms"
What is your differential diagnosis for her dyspareunia?
How would you evaluate her?
How would you address her climacteric symptoms?
What are alternatives to HRT?

3. "A 32-year-old female with hot flushes and amenorrhea for three months"
What is your differential diagnosis?
How would you evaluate her?
What treatment would you offer? (The answer ultimately was premature ovarian
failure.)

*Case list*

1. Bioidentical hormones—how do you counsel a patient?
2. Risks/benefits of HRT, with and without progesterone
3. What are the concerns with vaginal estrogen? If the patient now has vaginal
bleeding three months later, how would you work her up?
4. What is the mechanism for hot flushes? What are some non-hormonal options for
treatment?
5. Discussed other options for vasomotor symptoms besides hormonal therapy.

HRT—indications, contraindications, WHI study, counseling patients taking HRT(E&P) vs. ERT. The examiner wanted to me to state at what *age* do I terminate HRT. I tried the whole lowest dose and shortest duration, so I defended why I would continue therapy in 60+ and not *initiate* therapy.

## O. *Abnormal Uterine Bleeding

1. "A 38-year-old with menorrhagia-h/o menses x 10-14 days without BTB."
   Discuss etiologies, work-up (office biopsy vs. D&C), management (OCPs vs. proges-terone vs. D&C vs. hysterectomy vs. endometrial ablation, significance of atypia).

2. "A 13-year-old with LMP two weeks ago and a negative test for ßhCG has saturated pads every 30 minutes for the past two days."
   Discuss differential diagnosis, work-up, laboratory tests, treatment (including DDAVP). (Answer: Von Willibrands disease.

3. "A 39-year-old patient complains of intermenstrual spotting."
   Discuss differential diagnosis, evaluation
   "Sonohystogram reveals an echolucency."
   Discuss differential diagnosis, management, treatment (endometrial polyp).

4. "A 24-year-old 1G/0P whose LMP was seven weeks prior, presents with vaginal bleed-ing. Her HCG is 945."
   Discuss management.

5. "A patient has an HSG which demonstrates a submucosal fibroid."
   Discuss differential diagnosis, management, technique (including glycine hyponatremia).

6. "A 10-year-old presents with vaginal bleeding."
   Discuss differential diagnosis. (Answer: sarcoma botryroides.)

7. "A 15-year-old presents to ER after weeks of menorrhagia. She is orthostatic, and her Hct is 20."
   Define orthostasis and possible causes. What is your work-up? What labs would you order? What fluids would you give? Would you transfuse her? (No.) So the examiner made her Hct go down to 15
   Would you transfuse her? How would you treat her—IV vs. po? What type and dose of OCP?

8. "A patient complains of abnormal uterine bleeding. An exam reveals a mass prolapsing from the endocervical canal."
   What is your differential diagnosis?
   How would you evaluate her?
   If this is a prolapsing fibroid, describe your removal technique.

9. "A 4-year-old patient brought in by her parents with vaginal bleeding"
   What is your differential diagnosis?
   How would you work her up?
   How would you perform an exam?
   You see a tear in the labia majora on one side and purulent discharge from the vagina. What do you do now?

10. "Abnormal uterine bleeding in an adolescent."
    This became a brief discussion of AUB in patients of reproductive age, perimenopausal aged, and postmenopausal aged.

*Case List*
1. Mennorraghia work-up in a 14-, 23- ,45-, and 67-year-olds. As you can imagine, that went on for 10 minutes or so. (Several candidates had this.)
2. When do you sample a patient with a thickened endometrium?
3. W/U AUB in a 40-year-old vs. a 20-year-old
4. Management of submucosal fibroids

## P *Abnormal Cervical Cytology

1. <u>Abnormal Pap and Pregnancy</u>
   a. "A pregnant patient at 28 weeks EGA has a HGSIL Pap smear."
   Discuss counseling, evaluation, management (CIN III on cervical biopsy).

   b. Abnormal Pap and Pregnancy—"A 25-year-old 1G/0P has AGUS on her routine first trimester Pap smear."
   Discuss differential diagnosis, evaluation (including whether you would do an ECC), management (if micro-invasive).

2. <u>AGUS</u>
   a. "A 44-year-old with normal menses and a history of ASCUS, now presents with an AGUS Pap."
   Discuss work-up.
   "Would your management differ for a 19-year-old on OCPs or a 59-year-old menopausal patient?"

   b. "A 20-year-old with ASCUS Pap"
   How would you manage her? (Candidate responded repeat the Pap in one year.)
   "Okay, she's now 22 years old and has an ASCUS Pap, How would you manage her now?" (Candidate responded obtain reflex HPV.)
   "Her HPV is +. What now?" (Candidate responded he would perform colposcopy.)
   "Okay, she's now 15 years old and has an ASCUS with +HPV. What would you do?" (Candidate responded he would reprimand his office staff for ordering a HPV on a 15–year-old. The examiner laughed and moved on to a different topic.)

   c. "A 16-year-old with ASCUS Pap smear and + high risk HPV DNA"
   How would you manage her?
   "The repeat Pap smear next year is HGSIL."
   How would you manage her?
   "Her colposcopic directed biopsies show CIN 2."
   How would you manage her?

   d. "A 24-year-old with ASCUS Pap smear"
   How would you manage her?
   How does this change if her high risk HPV is +?
   What are her treatment options?

3. <u>CIN III</u>
   a. "A patient presents with recurrent CIN III."
   What would you do?

   b. "A 16-year-old with HSIL Pap"
   How would you manage her?
   How would your management change if she were a 21-year-old or a 41-year-old?
   How would you manage CIN II in either age group?

   c. "Patient with  HGSIL Pap smear"
   Describe your colposcopic technique.

4. <u>Post-hysterectomy Pap</u> – "A post-menopausal patient who is S/P TAH, BSO, and on HRT. A routine Pap shows ASCUS."
   Discuss work-up. How often would you perform a Pap if the hysterectomy was for benign/malignant disease?

5. <u>LEEP complications</u>
   a. "A patient presents to the ER with bleeding the evening after an office LEEP procedure."
      Discuss differential diagnosis, evaluation, management. What does LEEP stand for? Discuss your technique.

   b. "A patient is undergoing a LEEP procedure in the office and suddenly seizes."
      Discuss your differential diagnosis (Lidocaine toxicity), management (Lidocaine concentration, dosage), symptoms of Lidocaine toxicity.

   c. "A patient is undergoing an office LEEP procedure and has bleeding."
      What do you do?
      What measures could you have done to prevent?

   *Case List*

   1. 45-year-old who had a LEEP with involved margins. I had her booked for a hysterectomy, and the examiner wanted to know why. Also turned her into an adolescent and asked how my management would differ.
   2. Focused a lot on cervical cytology, Gardasil vaccine, how to manage abnormal Pap smear. One question pressed me on if I would offer the vaccine to someone who already had cervical dysplasia. I said yes, because if it was the quadravalent vaccine it would confer protection from other subtypes that the patient may not have been infected with.
   3. How would you manage bleeding for a LEEP conducted in the office?
   4. Heavy emphasis on Pap triage and focus on new clinical guidelines.
   5. HGSIL—management and follow-up: changed age from 30 to 20 years.
   6. They asked me, "How do you do a colposcopy? What is the mechanism of acetic acid? What is the management of a LEEP or CKC if you have positive margins? How do you counsel your patients about LEEP vs. Cone? When do you do a CKC? When do you do a LEEP?"
   7. A patient had a LEEP with involved margins. I had her booked for a hysterectomy, and the examiner wanted to know why. Also turned her into an adolescent and asked how my management would differ

## Q. Vaginal Discharge

"A 42-year-old, who uses condoms, develops a watery vaginal discharge after intercourse and c/o vaginal discomfort."
   Discuss differential diagnosis (infectious and non-infectious) wet mount, pH.

*Case List*

"You treated this patient with Diflucan for her yeast. How would you manage her if she has recurrent symptoms?" (Candidate responded to treat with Terazol.) "The patient is no better. What now?" (Candidate got a fungal culture.) "The fungal culture grows *Candida gelabrata*. How do you treat her now?" (Candidate responded, "With boric acid.)

### R. Vulvar Disease

1. Hidradenitis suppurativa of vulva with drainage tracts—"A patient complains of reoccurring vulvar pimples. Exam reveals multiple boils with sinuses."
   Discuss, evaluation, management (including medical and surgical).

2. Vulvar dystrophy—"A 60-year-old presents with vulvar pruritis."
   Discuss differential diagnosis, work-up, treatment.

3. Necrotizing fasciitis—"A diabetic patient presents to your office two days after a vulvar biopsy with a foul-smelling discharge from the biopsy site."
   Discuss differential diagnosis (necrotizing fasciitis), work-up, management, microbiology, antibiotic selection.

3. Skin cancer—"A patient presents with a lesion on the skin."
   Discuss evaluation. Treatment if basal cell vs. squamous cell cancer vs. malignant melanoma.

4. Lichens planus
   a. "An elderly lady with vulvar lesion typical of lichen planus"
   How do you decide when to biopsy?
   How would you treat her and for how long?
   How do you follow up?
   "A 20-something-year-old lady with vulvar lesion"
   What is your differential diagnosis?
   How would you manage her?
   When does she follow up?

5. Vulvar ulcers—"A 26-year-old woman presents with a vulval ulcer"
   What is your differential diagnosis?
   How will you evaluate her?
   How will you treat?

6. Bartholin's—"A 41-year-old with a 3cm mass inside introitus"
   What is your differential diagnosis?
   "Patient is determined she has a Bartholin's abscess"
   How would you manage her? (Candidate: I&D and placed a Word catheter.)
   "Her Word catheter falls out and she returns the next day. What now?"
   What determines whether you I&D vs. marsupialization vs. excision?

   *Case List*

   1. What is your differential diagnosis for a worrisome mole? If the biopsy shows malignant melanoma, how would you manage her? (Candidate referred, so the examiner responded with, "What would your consultant do?")
   2. "How do you manage a patient if she does not respond to treatment for lichens sclerosus?" (Candidate replied to perform a biopsy). "The biopsy returns VIN3." How would you treat her?
   3. Discussed treatment of Bartholin's cyst for a 23-year-old vs. a 47-year-old female.

### R. Urinary/Fecal Incontinence and Pelvic Floor Defects

1. Prolapse
   a. "An 89-year-old nursing home resident is brought to your office with procidentia with ulceration.
   Discuss management, counseling.
   "Family refuses pessary"
   Discuss surgical options.
   Discuss how your approach changes if she is a 59-year-old.

    b.  "Patient had a TAH years ago. Now presents with a bulge in the vagina."
       What is your differential diagnosis?
       How do you evaluate her? (Diagnosis ends up being an enterocele.)
       How do you repair an enterocele?
       Can you do anything to prevent it?

    c.  "How do you avoid damaging the bladder and ureters in a patient who is undergoing surgery for procidentia?"

## 2. Urinary Incontinence

"A woman (cannot remember age) presents with a complaint of losing urine."
What is your differential diagnosis?
How would you evaluate her?

## 3. Fecal Incontinence

    a.  "A patient presents three months post partum passing flatus through the vagina."
       Discuss differential diagnosis, work-up.
       "Physical exam shows no obvious defect."
       What now?

    b.  Episiotomy breakdown—"A patient presents one week post partum with broken down fourth degree episiotomy repair."
       Discuss management.

    c.  "A patient is six weeks from an SVD and presents with complaints of passage of stool and gas from the vagina."
       What is your differential diagnosis?
       How would you evaluate her?
       When would you repair a rectovaginal fistula?
       Describe your surgical technique for the repair of a rectovaginal fistula.
       Are there any preoperative considerations?
       What is your postoperative management?

    d.  "A 44-year-old G4P4 complains of passing stool and flatus per vagina."
       What is the differential diagnosis?
       How would you work her up? (PE is normal except you notice decreased sphincter tone.)
       How would you treat?
       "A 24-year-old after a vaginal delivery with the above complaints"
       Diagnosis and management of rectovaginal fistula.
       What percent heal spontaneously?
       What does conservative treatment consist of?

    e.  "A 38-year-old, S/P NSVD 10 years ago, presents with fecal incontinence."
       What are common causes? (Although I just studied this, I could only think of obstetric injury, trauma, neurological/motor problem.)
       How do you evaluate? (I focused on my history and physical for a while. I described in detail, looking for the dovetail sign, bulbocavernous reflex, etc. I ordered an anal U/S, EMG, and Anal manometry depending on patient's history and sensory capabilities. I had to explain how the anal U/S would help delineate a defect in the external anal sphincter vs. internal anal sphincter.
       Then the examiner asked me to evaluate a 20-something-year-old female S/P NSVD two weeks prior with incontinence of stool and flatus.
       What is your differential diagnosis?
       How to evaluate? (So again, I focused on H&P, especially the obstetric history.)
       Then the examiner asked to me to compare and contrast the two patients regarding my differential, evaluation, and treatment. (I stated I would delay

treatment in the postpartum patient because there's most likely a wound break-down in the 3/4 degree repair with evidence of infection/edema. I stated I would give antibiotics, stool softener, low residue diet, etc., and delay surgery for 2-3 months. [I remember this case because I was like **why me??!!**])

## S. Urinary Tract Infections

1. Recurrent UTIs—"A 23-year-old with recurrent UTIs and negative cervical cultures."
   Discuss work-up, management, suppression.

2. UTI
   a. "A patient with a history of a kidney problem at age 3 now presents with a positive urinalysis."
      Discuss differential diagnosis, work-up (including protein, BUN/creatinine), management.

   b. "A 30-year-old calls at 2 am with dysuria, frequency"
      How do you evaluate?
      Would you phone in a prescription for empiric treatment or would you send her to the ED?

3. Nephrolithiasis—"A 54-year-old 3G/2P, who recently stopped her HRT and is now taking 4g of calcium a day, presents with acute right flank pain and night lower abdominal pain."
   Discuss differential diagnosis, evaluation. (Answer: kidney stone.) Management, counseling.

4. "A 40-year-old with asymptomatic bacteriuria"
   Indications for treatment

5. "A patient c/o dysuria, UA +nitrites, otherwise negative.
   What is your differential diagnosis? (Candidate responded HSV, vaginitis, interstitial cystitis, condom latex allergy.)

## T. *Sexually Transmitted Diseases (STDs)

1. Vulvar ulcers

   a. "A patient presents with a painful vesicular lesion on her vulva."
      Discuss differential diagnosis, work-up, treatment.

   b. "A 20-year-old virgin with painful ulcerative lesion on vulva following oral sex"
      Differential diagnosis?
      Diagnostic approach?
      Management options?

2. Syphilis
   "A 24-year-old with a positive VDRL, performed after she complained of having had a lesion on her vulva."
   Discuss counseling, work-up, treatment.

3. PID
   "After a TAH, BSO for a tubo-ovarian abscess, the patient has nausea and vomiting."
   Discuss differential diagnosis, evaluation. What IVFs would you give? What if her potassium was 2.8?
   "After 6 days of conservative management, she has not improved."
   What do you do? What tests do you order?
   "A CT scan shows a fluid collection of 8cm."
   How do you proceed?

"A KUB shows air/fluid levels and bowel wall edema."
What do you do?
"When repairing a circular hole in the bowel, which direction should the repair be?"
Which suture would you use for which layer?

B. Management for
"A patient with Gonorrhea"
"A patient with Chlamydia"
"A patient with +RPR"

*Case List*

"If a patient has a + Chlamydia culture, what other STDs would you screen for?"
Would you perform a test of cure?

## U. Pediatric Gynecology

## V. Sexual Assault, Spousal Abuse

1. <u>Battered women, chronic pelvic pain</u>—"A patient is accompanied by her husband to your office. He informs you she has had pelvic pain for months. You note multiple bruises." Discuss work-up, management.

2. <u>Sexual assault</u>
   a. "A 21-year-old, 10-14 days after her LMP, presents to the emergency room four hours after being raped." Discuss methods of collecting specimens and evidence, work-up, counseling, emergency contraception (protocol, effectiveness, follow-up), STD screen, and prophylaxis.

   b. "A patient was assaulted 3 days ago and presents to your office."
   Discuss your state's regulations and how you would collect evidence. Discuss laboratory evaluation, HIV prophylaxis, STD treatment.
   "Physical exam reveals tear posterior fourchette vs. high up in posterior fornix." Discuss management (exploratory laparotomy if a fornix injury

## U. PMS, PMDD, Depression
1. <u>PMS/PMDD</u>
   a. "A patient complains of irritability, bloating, depression during luteal phase." Discuss diagnosis (symptom calendar) and management (referral for severe depression and/or suicidal thoughts).

   b. "A patient complains of decreased interest one week prior to her menses." What is your differential diagnosis?
   "Her complaints are now daily and affecting her quality of life." How would you treat her?
   What medications would you use?
   What medications would you use is she desires a pregnancy?

2. <u>Depression</u>
   a. "A woman presents c/o fatigue and weight loss."
   Discuss differential diagnosis, evaluation, treatment.

   b. "A postmenopausal patient complains of depression, anxiety, and fatigue" What is your differential diagnosis?
   How would you evaluate her?
   How would you treat her?
   What medications would you use?

3. Anxiety—"A patient c/o fatigue, insomnia, anxiety and irritability."
Discuss differential diagnosis, evaluation, treatment

*Case List*

PMS—How do you diagnose it? What medications do you use?

## V. Benign Pelvic Masses

"Patient with pelvic pain"
What is your differential diagnosis? (Ends up with an ovarian mass.)
How would you work up the mass?
What tumor markers would you obtain?
Asked same questions but changed age from teen to reproductive age to
menopause

## W. Ultrasound

I got grilled about the ultrasounds that I said I did and what sort of
quality assurance measures we have for our ultrasounds, and on and on.
Not totally sure what they were looking for there.

## X. Back Pain

1. Arthritis—"A patient presents with arthritis."
Discuss types of arthritis, work-up, management.

2. "Patient using NSAIDs develops peripheral edema."
Patient ultimately went on to acute renal failure and upper GI bleeding.

3. Sciatica

4. Herniated disc

## Y. Respiratory Tract Diseases

Tuberculosis

## Z. Gastrointestinal Diseases

Peptic ulcer disease—Differential diagnosis, treatment, most common cause (*H. pylori*)

## AA. Cardiovascular Diseases

1. CVA— "A 61-year-old female calls from home, c/o slurred speech and dizziness for the
past 20 minutes."
What would you do?
Would you advise her to come to the office or ER?

2. CV—"A patient in pre-op holding c/o chest pain."
Discuss differential diagnosis, work-up. (Answer: acute myocardial infarction.)

3. Coumadin
   a. "A patient with atrial fibrillation on Coumadin needs a hysterectomy."
   How do you transition her from Coumadin to Heparin and back after surgery?
   How do you run a Heparin drip?

b. "A 63-year-old patient with a history of atrial fibrillation on Coumadin requires a D&C/hysterectomy for post-menopausal bleeding."
What are the issues with her anti-coagulation and her upcoming surgery?
How do you decide whether she needs to stop her Coumadin or transition to Heparin?
Discuss how you counsel the patient in this transition.
Discuss risks, complications, monitoring, and mechanism of action for both Coumadin and Heparin.

## BB. Hypertension

* Hypertension, hyperlipidemia—"Healthy, postmenopausal woman presents for her annual exam with BP of 170/120 mmHg."
Discuss diagnosis of hypertension, definition of essential hypertension, medications, screening for concurrent diseases.

## CC. Dyslipidemia

1. *Dyslipidemia—"A 30-year-old with a total cholesterol of 240 and an LDL 160" or "a 39-year-old with diabetes, G/P TAH, BSO on ERT has an LDL 190."
Discuss evaluation, risks for CVD, management (including diet, exercise, and medications). Would you discontinue her ERT? If so, what alternatives would you offer her?

2. "An 18-year-old, obese, on OCP with elevated triglyceride level"
Differential diagnosis for hypertriglyceridemia
Management options

3. "A patient with hypercholesterolemia"
What labs do you order?
When do you refer?
What medications are available for treatment?

## DD. Substance Abuse

## EE. Other

1. Headaches—"A patient presents c/o chronic headaches."
Discuss differential diagnosis, evaluation, management (migraines vs. tension headache), influence of HRT.

2. Vaginal mass—"What type of cysts would you find in the vagina?"
Discuss differential diagnosis. (Answer: Bartholin's cyst.) Management for a 20-year-old vs. a 50-year-old.

3. Anemia—"Elderly female presents with weakness and dizziness."
Discuss differential diagnosis (anemia), work-up (GI bleed), colonoscopy (negative, but hemoccult positive). What next?

# 8

## Chapter

# Studying for the Exam

The focus of this book until now has been the individualized study strategy applied to specific phases of preparation for the oral exam. This chapter addresses the process of studying in general.

You must first prioritize your study topics. Ideally, this is accomplished about six months before the exam, when you attend your first review course. Your objective in prioritizing is to identify and rank your personal strengths and weaknesses across the range of study topics that are covered during the review course. Compare this list with topics that you know will be on the exam. Know cold the topics in Table 1 (next page), which have occurred time and time again and are virtually guaranteed to appear on your exam. The "hot topics" in Table 2 occur frequently but not as often as the "know cold" topics. Kodachromes and case-of-the-day lists obtained from candidate recall from past exams can be found in Chapters 6 and 7, respectively.

Combine the above lists, and draft an updated priority list. Stash it away for later reference. Next, funnel all your energy into compiling the case list. After the case list is cast in stone, identify the study topics that it generates. Cross-reference this study list with the earlier list generated above. Once again, compare the two lists and prioritize an updated list.

Dedicate one month of study, typically two months before your exam, to learning your case list cold. You should cover the majority of topics generated by your case list. Add the remaining topics into the topic list drafted earlier, and once again reprioritize an updated study list. Your remaining time should be spent whittling away at the list. Some additional topics may be generated by mock oral exams. With only one month to go, accept that it is impossible to cover the entire list. Reprioritize the remaining topics every week.

Stop in-depth studying one week before the exam. Spend the last week simply reviewing this mass of information. Solidify your strengths. Polish your articulation of this knowledge with mock oral exams. Refer to the end of the chapter for specific guidelines on how to make the most of this critical study aid. It's simply not good enough for this exam to be only book smart.

### TABLE 1   "Know Cold" Topics

#### I. Obstetrics

1. Shoulder dystocia: risk factors and management (including algorithm of maneuvers)

2. Breech presentation: delivery route debate, cardinal maneuvers for vaginal delivery, external cephalic version, twin breech extraction

3. Postpartum hemorrhage—risk factors, differential diagnosis, stabilization, management: uterotonics (types, mechanism of action, contraindications, dose, duration), surgical management (O'Leary uterine artery ligation, B-Lynch suture, hemostatic square suture, hypogastric artery ligation, cesarean hysterectomy), uterine artery embolization, blood replacement

#### II. Gynecology

1. Ureter: anatomic course, sites of injury, injury recognition and management, injury prevention

2. Procidentia: work-up and surgical approach, especially sacrospinous ligament fixation, prevention

3. Stress urinary incontinence: work-up (standing stress test, Q-tip test), differentiation from urge incontinence, management (surgical vs. conservative), surgical technique, management of intra- and/or post-operative complications

4. Hysterectomy: alternatives, selection of route, intra- and/or post-operative complications; vaginal hysterectomy: surgical technique, candidates, laparoscopic candidates

#### III. Office Practice

1. Adnexal mass: influence of age, differential diagnosis, work-up

2. Amenorrhea: presentation, differential diagnosis, work-up, treatment

3. Preventive care and health maintenance per age group: schedule for Pap smears, mammograms, colorectal, BMD screening, laboratory tests, immunizations

4. Contraception: counseling, types, indications/contraindications, mechanism of action, complications

5. Polycystic ovarian syndrome (PCOS): presentation, work-up (labs, imaging), cause, treatment (OCPs, progesterone, GnRH agonists—mechanism of action, dosing, side effects), associated metabolic syndrome, hirsutism (pharmacologic and local treatment)

## IV. Other

1. Drugs: brand and generic name, components (especially for OCPs and HRT), mechanism of action, indications/contraindications, administration (dose, duration), side effects, antidote

2. Labs: units, effect of timing

---

## TABLE 2    "Hot Topics" on the Oral Exam

## I. Obstetrics

1. Vaginal birth after cesarean section (VBAC): candidates, contraindications, counseling risks/benefits, labor management, recognition/management of uterine rupture

2. Hypertensive disorders of pregnancy: definitions (gestational HTN, chronic HTN, preeclampsia (severe), eclampsia), diagnosis, work-up, antepartum management, timing for delivery, intrapartum management (MgSO4, anti-hypertensives) HELLP syndrome, DIC

3. Group B beta streptococci (GBS): screening, risk factors, management, antibiotics (selection, options if PCN allergic, timing)

4. Diabetes mellitus: Pre-existing (preconception counseling, associated congenital anomalies), gestational diabetes mellitus (GDM) screening, diagnosis, antenatal vs. labor management, fetal management at delivery, macrosomia

5. Isoimmunization, nonimmune hydrops: recognition, management, Lilly curve, RhoGAM

6. Post dates: definition, management (when and how to induce)

7. Labor dysfunction: Friedman labor curve: be able to draw (especially if failure-to-progress terminology is used on your case list), diagnosis, management

8. Prolonged rupture of membranes: when to induce

9. Preterm rupture of membranes: effect of gestational age on management, organisms, antibiotics, diagnosis of chorioamnionitis

10. Forceps vs. vacuum: outlet vs. low vs. mid, indications for each, how long to pull, types of fetal trauma

11. Induction of labor: cervical ripening, Pitocin protocols, IUPCs

12. Preterm labor: risk factors, causes, management (steroids, tocolytics, fetal fibronectin), management in subsequent pregnancy (17-OH progesterone, cervical length, fetal fibronectin)

13. Intrauterine growth retardation: symmetric vs. asymmetric, causes

14. Multifetal pregnancy: chorion/amnion status (diagnosis, clinical significance), twin-to-twin transfusion (diagnosis, management), antepartum management, presentation and delivery options

15. Bleeding in pregnancy: first-trimester vs. second-trimester vs. third-trimester

    a. Placenta abruption: risk factors, diagnosis, antepartum/intrapartum management (DIC, blood replacement)

    b. Placenta previa/accreta: risk factors, diagnosis, antepartum management, intraoperative management, complications/sequale

16. Dating of pregnancy: LMP vs. Neagle's rule vs. ultrasound vs. serial HCGs

17. Thromboembolic disorders: risk factors, especially inheritable, work-up, prophylaxis, diagnosis and management (including heparin, how molecular weight heparin, Coumadin) of DVT and pulmonary embolus

18. Infections: HIV, Hepatitis, TORCH, Syphilis, Rubella, Varicella, Parvovirus: recognition, work-up, management—ante- vs. intra- vs. postpartum, fetal effects

19. Fetal distress: recognition on FHR monitor strips, differential diagnosis of causes, management (including amnioinfusion)

20. Antepartum testing: non-stress test, contraction stress test, biophysical profile

21. Preconception counseling: counseling options—CVS, amniocentesis, ultrasound, soft markers, maternal serum screening (components of, sensitivity/specificity, further work-up)

22. Episiotomy: routine vs. indicated, type—midline vs. mediolateral, complications —3$^{rd}$, 4$^{th}$ repair

23. Cesarean delivery: maternal request—counseling; multiple repeats—antepartum management, counseling, intraoperative management including cesarean hysterectomy

## II. Gynecology

1. Abnormal uterine bleeding (AUB): definition DUB, causes, work-up—and influence of age, management (including ablation)

2. Hysteroscopy: counseling, technique, diagnostic vs. operative (distending media, management of I/O discrepancy)

3. Leiomyomata: symptoms, evaluation, treatment (medical vs. hysteroscopic vs. embolization) vs. surgical—selection of route of hysterectomy, pre- and intraoperative measures to decrease bleeding

4. Pelvic inflammatory disease: causative organisms, presentation, outpatient vs. inpatient management, antibiotics, surgical management

5. Sterilization: counseling, types (hysteroscopic occlusion, postpartum, laparoscopic), laparoscopic tubal ligation: failure, technique, issues for reversal, anesthesia risks

6. Oncology, especially cervical, ovarian, uterine: presentation, work-up, when to refer, when to stage

7. Endometrial hyperplasia: significance of atypia, office endometrial sampling vs. D&C, hormonal vs. surgical treatment, uterine cancer

8. Abnormal cervical cytology: role of HPV, Gardasil, influence of age on management, ASCUS, AGUS, colposcopy technique and interpretation, LEEP vs. CKC, management of involved margins

9. Ectopic pregnancy: work-up, diagnosis (ultrasound, HCGs), medical management (candidates, methotrexate—mechanism of action, dosing, surveillance, complications), surgical management (laparoscopy vs. laparotomy, salpingectomy vs. salpingostomy)

10. Laparoscopy: technique, safety, types of injury (GI, vascular, ureter)

11. Blood replacement therapy: indications, PRBCs, FFP, cyroprecipitate

12. Thromboembolic disorders: risk factors, especially inheritable, work-up, prophylaxis, diagnosis and management (including Heparin, low molecular weight Heparin, Coumadin) of DVT and pulmonary embolus

13. Bladder injuries: prevention, recognition; intraoperative vs. postoperative; management— intraoperative and postoperative, duration of drainage

13. Gastrointestinal injuries: prevention, recognition, management of bowel injury (intra- and postoperative: SBO vs. ileus—work-up, radiologic findings, management)

14. Post-op wound complications: recognition (seroma, cellulites, dehiscence, evisceration), management

15. Post-op fever: differential diagnosis, work-up, management

16. Endometriosis: pathophysiology, presentation, work-up, medical management (OCPs, progesterone, GnRH agonists), surgical management (intraoperative findings, approach), postoperative management

17. Chronic pelvic pain: differential diagnosis, work up, treatment

18. Adnexal mass: differential diagnosis, work-up (influence of age, tumor markers), management (influence of size, imaging features suggestive of benign vs. malignancy)

19. Peri-operative coexisting medical problems (respiratory, cardiac, diabetes, electrolyte disturbances, anticoagulation): screening, work-up, when to get preoperative clearance, when to postpone surgery, management of medications (Coumadin, oral hypoglycemics, insulin, anti-hypertensives), postoperative complications, life-threatening problem management

## III. Office Practice

1. Abnormal lactation: presentation, work-up (labs, MRI, x-ray), treatment, management in pregnancy

2. Primary/secondary amenorrhea: presentation, work-up (including congenital abnormalities: Mayer-Rokitansky-Kuster-Hauser Syndrome, testicular feminization, Turner's ), causes, treatment

3. Precocious and delayed puberty: normal puberty, definitions, causes, work up, treatment

4. Breast disease:

   a. breast lump – physical exam, work-up, breast cyst aspiration (technique, what to do depending upon type of aspirate—bloody, golden, green, dry aspirate) management, when to refer

   b. breast discharge – physical exam, work-up and management, depending upon type of discharge—milky, bloody, clear, green, golden

5. Chronic pelvic pain: differential diagnosis, work-up

6. Basic infertility: up to and including treatment with Clomid

7. Premenstrual dysphoric disorder (PMDD), PMS, Depression: diagnosis, treatment (medications, alternatives)

8. Ambiguous genitalia (congenital adrenal hyperplasia): normal sexual development, presentation, work-up, causes, definitions

9. STDs: vulvar ulcer work up, Syphilis, Gonorrhea, Chlamydia, Hepatitis B, C, HIV, Herpes, PID: presentation, causative organism, CDC antibiotics

10. Primary care: screening, diagnosis, initial management, criteria for referral

    a. HTN – diagnosis, definition, anti-hypertensive medications

    b. Diabetes – screening, diagnosis, medications (oral vs. insulin)

    c. Thyroid disease (hyper- and hypo-)—presentation, work-up (labs), treatment (thyroid replacement, PTU)

    d. Dyslipidemia—screening (labs), treatment (medications, alternatives)

    e. Gastrointestinal disease—chronic constipation, irritable bowel syndrome, diarrhea, dyspepsia, PUD

    f. Respiratory tract disease—asthma, community acquired pneumonia, tuberculosis

11. Menopause: HRT (risks vs. benefits; defense of your drug preference; knowledge of specific hormone content), WHI study

12. Osteoporosis: risk factors, bone density ( interpretation, Z vs. T score), treatment

13. Endometriosis: pathogenesis, presentation, work-up, medical management (OCPs, progesterone, GnRH agonists)

14. Abnormal Pap smear (ASCUS, AGUS, SIL): work-up (high-risk HPV DNA), treatment

15. Obesity: BMI, counseling, treatment (medications and alternatives)

16. Smoking cessation: counseling, treatment

17. Substance abuse: recognition, counseling, work-up

18. Sexual dysfunction: types, counseling, treatment

19. Vulvar disease: differential diagnosis chancre, vulvar dystrophy, skin cancer (malignant melanoma)

22. Urinary incontinence, overactive bladder: work-up, treatment (medical vs. bladder training), stress urinary incontinence, Kegel exercises

23. Prolapse: pessaries

24. Sexual assault: state reporting requirements, collection or evidence, STD testing and treatment, emergency contraception, counseling

25. Intimate partner violence: recognition, counseling (escape plan), state reporting requirements

---

Another means by which to study topics is through reviewing gross and microscopic pathology. Historically, these were an integral part of the test but were deleted as a specific component in the mid 1990s. Until 1997, the ABOG *Bulletin* stated that interpretation of "gross and microscopic pathology" was fair game. However, subsequent *Bulletins* eliminated this specific wordage and replaced it with "interpretation of sonograms, operating videos and videographics of various conditions."

Currently, a rare Kodachrome of a gross or microscopic pathology specimen has appeared on the exam. Even if you don't recognize it, the examiner will tell you the diagnosis without penalty. What is important is to be able to discuss the evaluation and management of the disease process. For the sake of completeness, I have included, in Table 3 below, the list of slides that traditionally appeared when interpretation of microscopic slides was a required exam component. Time is precious. I would not prioritize the study of pathology. I dare say, I wouldn't study them at all.

**TABLE 3**   Past Pathology Microscopic Slides

---

**1. Fallopian tube**

- Salpingitis
- Salpingitis isthmica nodosa
- Ectopic pregnancy

**2. Vagina**

- Adenosis
- Clear cell adenocarcinoma

**3. Vulva**

- VIN III
- Vulvar dystrophy; lichen sclerosus and squamous hyperplasia
- Papillary hidradenoma

- Squamous cell carcinoma
- Extramammary Paget's disease
- Condylomata

**4. Cervix**
- Sqaumous cell carcinoma
- HGSIL
- Condylomata

**5. Uterus**
- Leiomyomata
- Adenomyosis
- Proliferative endometrium
- Complex adenomatous hyperplasia vs. atypia
- Adenocarcinoma
- Hydatidiform mole

**6. Ovary**
- Mudinous cystadenoma or cystadenocarcinoma
- Serous cystadenoma or cystadenocarcinoma
- Brenner's tumor
- Dysgerminoma
- Granulosa cell
- Mature cystic tertoma
- Endometriosis

---

In conclusion, you must have a written study plan. Prioritize the subjects based upon exam probability, personal strengths and weaknesses, and topics generated by your case list. Reevaluate your plan as needed, and draft an updated plan accordingly. Confine your study to a clinically oriented review. Acknowledge that it is impossible to study everything on your list. Finally, don't forget to take breaks to avoid burnout.

## Mock Oral Exams

You can study all you want, but if you can't articulate what you know, then you simply will not pass this test. I have met a rare individual who can pull this off without practice, but most of you will procrastinate, delaying the inevitable until the last minute. Why would you spend a year collecting cases, study for months, and then scrimp on undergoing mock oral exams, the most important study tool of all?

I have mentored candidates preparing for their oral board exam for nearly twenty years. Usually it takes only three mock oral exams for most to become comfortable with this mode of examination. Just like any new skill, the learning curve is exponential.

First, let's give credit where credit is due. Admit it: you simply could not have made it this far if you were not pretty clever. Come on, you made it through MCATs, medical school, USMLEs, residency, CREOG in-service training exams, and the written boards. You are one smart dude/gal. However, what was the most common test format for all of these? Yup, that's right, the written exam. So trust me on this one. You must take some mock oral exams. You will be ever so glad you did. Now let me show you how.

First, let's start with the one examiner to whom you have ready access …namely **you**! Don't underestimate yourself at all. As a matter of fact, you will be the toughest person to get past. I conduct oral exam workshops, and right away, we put you in the examiner's seat. Everyone comments about how they totally underestimated how helpful another candidate can be.

You are helpful in two ways. First look at your or another candidate's case list. What would you ask if you were the examiner? At the workshop, the most popular session is when we allow you to present your nightmare case. Everyone gets to fire any possible question her or she foresees. We have determined it takes just six to eight minutes to flush out all questions. Hands down, the questions that were predicted in this session were indeed asked on the actual exam.

Secondly, quiz yourself out loud. Refer back to those "know cold" topics that we discussed earlier in this chapter, such as a vaginal breech delivery. Write out the management on an index card and rote memorize the answer. You can post these on your bathroom mirror, take them with you in the car on your commute, or review them when you exercise.

Now practice out loud alone. You must get familiar with answering out loud, rather than silently. Unfortunately, you don't sound nearly as eloquent out loud as you do in your head.

Now practice in front of the mirror. **Yikes!** Would you trust that guy delivering your vaginal breech? Practice until the answer is a resounding yes.

Okay, now involve your loved ones. You really need their support during this trying time. They will so much more supportive if you enlist their aid. Practice your rote answer with your spouse. They don't need to know a darn thing about a vaginal breech delivery. However, it is ever so helpful to use another person as a sounding board. Give them your index cards, so they can follow along. They will readily note if you left anything out.

Let's stay in your comfort zone. Next enlist your partner or another colleague's help. At this point, you don't have to make a big deal out it. Just ask them to listen to your answer as you are closing on an abdominal case or in the doctor's lounge in between cases.

Finally, now it's time to schedule some mock oral exams to practice defending your case list. No, this is not a review and troubleshoot of anticipated topics, but an actual mock oral exam. That means you need to use the case list that you submitted to ABOG; yes, the one that lacks all your crib notes. I strongly advocate tapping into some local and regional colleagues. There is a tendency to procrastinate as you will feel you are not ready. Yet you will probably never be ready if you go by your standards. Besides, you don't want to be embarrassed by acknowledging you don't know everything.

Guess what? Your colleagues already know you don't know everything, because they don't either! Remember, you are at your knowledge peak. You will probably never know so much about so much again. So give yourself a break and just dive on in. I guarantee not one, not a single colleague, will decline your request to give you a mock oral exam. It is an honor to help another colleague.

So what are some examples of local and regional colleagues? Local colleagues are those right there in your community where you practice. This would include partners in your group, those that you share call with, or other generalists in your town.

Regional colleagues are typically those subspecialists that you refer to. This is a great opportunity to get to know them, since most of the time you're communicating by phone. In addition, remember your examiner will most likely be a subspecialist, so it is nice to get that perspective, especially if you are a generalist. So have your referring MFM quiz you on your obstetrics case list, your GYN oncologist on your gynecology list, and your REI on your office and gynecology case list.

Your local and regional colleagues are plentiful, readily available, and at the right price, but you get what you pay for. If they do not routinely give mock oral exams, then their only experience will most likely be their own oral board exam. An $n = 1$ in any study is of very limited value, so give them the following guidelines and instructions so they can effectively help you practice.

1. Ideally review my case list ahead of time and pick out the top ten cases.

2. Let's start with those top ten cases. You can tell me later why those were of interest to you.

3. Do you mind if I record this? Here, let me quickly set up the camcorder. Don't worry, I've got it aimed on me, but my wife/husband/partner tells me I have this crazy nervous tic. I want to see for myself. Besides, even though I know you, I still get nervous, and I can't remember the questions and responses for later review.

4. I brought a stop clock. Let's go for ten minutes straight, then later twenty, then ultimately for thirty minutes, as on the test.

5. I really appreciate your help, but do not interrupt to give me feedback. We'll do that after our designated time.

6. You're going to love this, but don't be nice to me. It doesn't help at all. Put on your best poker face. No feedback, no encouragement, no smiling, no nodding of the head, no nothing.

7. Please write down my answers. That will help to keep us both on track with the line of questioning; plus it simulates the exam. I can also refer to your notes when I review the taped recording.

Another pool of mock oral examiners is academicians, including those past and present. Call the residency director of the closest residency. I'm sure either he and/or his faculty would be happy to help you out. Why not make a trip back to where you did your residency and meet with your residency director or some of your favorite faculty? Better yet, choose that one faculty member that was always so tough on you. Yeah, the jerk ... he's perfect. Don't assume that they have experience in mock oral exams. Remember, they were preparing you for the written boards. You may need to give them the above guidelines too.

Finally, I recommend you take at least one mock oral exam with a professional. This is someone who is remunerated for providing this service, so is typically a faculty member from a review or tutorial course. Do not assume that just because he/she is being paid that he/she is qualified. Verify his/her credentials, experience, and track record, especially if he/she is a clinician. A past board examiner is the ultimate, unless of course he/she is no longer practicing medicine.

After you have taken a few mock oral exams, you will appreciate the tricks your mind can play. The biggest and final obstacle to overcome is **you**. If you truly believe you will pass this exam, then you will. Believe in yourself!

Mind your mind. Envision the whole process, starting with your arrival in Dallas. Put your suit on, look at yourself and emblazon the image in your mind. Now put yourself in the exam room. Envision the examiners and you answering their questions thoughtfully, confidently, and quickly. Set yourself up for success. Make it so!

In conclusion, you cannot attempt this exam unprepared. You have to be book smart, but you must be able to articulate persuasively this knowledge. I suppose any old mock oral exam is better than no mock oral exam. However, you will excel quicker if you give your mock oral examiners guidelines on how to help you best. Practice doesn't make perfect. Rather, *perfect practice* makes perfect. Practice for the real thing. Anything less is second best.

# 9

# Image Enhancement

Y ou can't judge a book by its cover—or can you? Image enhancement is a facet of testmanship that traditionally has often been ignored. Image enhancement refers to the strategy of optimizing not what you say, but how you say it. In other words, it is how to influence positively or manipulate the examiner's first impression.

Stereotypically, physicians ignore society's emphasis on the physical impression, whereas in other professions (such as business or law) one's image can make or break a deal or case. A well-known study concluded that the first impression is based predominantly (55%) on appearance. The quality of one's voice, such as tone, pitch, and speech pattern, has a 38% influence, with a mere 7% is based on what you say. Furthermore, the first impression is made within only five seconds.

Some of you may argue that you don't have to, that you don't want to, and ultimately that you refuse to play the game. But given all the effort that has gone into preparing for this exam, can you really afford not to? Why not approach this issue as stacking the deck? Not bucking the system but beating the system. Besides, if you don't like the system, then change it when *you're* the examiner. Remember, "You can't change the system if you're not in the system."

Testmanship is knowing not only what is on the exam, but who the examiner is. An examiner's academic profile influences the type of questions that he or she asks. Similarly, understanding the examiner's physical image will give you yet another insight into his or her makeup. The more you know about the examiners, the better armed you are to battle with them.

Most examiners are leaders in their field. This status usually dictates frequent public and peer exposure and hence conformity to a stereotypic dress code. The majority of the examiners have been middle-aged males. However, increasingly more examiners are women. Stereotypically, all examiners dress conservatively. Typical attire for a male examiner is khaki pants, a navy sport coat, and a button-down shirt with a bow tie or a paisley or striped tie. A female examiner will be similarly conservatively attired in a pant suit or skirt.

I want to reiterate the importance of the first impression that your case list makes. Remember, the examiner has already reviewed your case list before he meets you. The mental image he has of you is based solely on your case list. When the examiner actually meets you, he or she will quickly see if the impression matches. This is the time—and you only have five seconds—either to solidify a positive impression or persuade the examiner to reconsider if he or she has misjudged you.

Let's now walk through the components involved in the first five critical seconds with the examiner. The most influential is appearance. The two most important components of appearance are tailoring and color. Tailoring should capitalize on your positive physical features and downplay the negative. For example, if you are overweight, choose clothes that make you look more lean. Simply lengthening the tie distracts from a protuberant abdomen. I recommend that men wear a suit and tie. A sport coat, although collegiate, is not as professional as a two-piece suit.

For women, the theme is conservative yet feminine and fashionable clothes. Appropriate attire is either a dress or a two-piece suit (pant or skirt). A skirt or pants and blouse without a jacket is too plain and not as professional.

Color can make an impact, either negative or positive. An inexpensive investment that lasts a lifetime is to have your colors professionally analyzed. Many companies offer a trained image consultant who, with the help of computer analysis, can determine your most complimentary colors. Extensive research is available to determine what impact certain colors will make.

Safe colors for your suit are blue, black and brown. Grey, which is a common color, is rarely flattering for most, unless you have black or grey hair. A suit that matches your hair color makes the whole package flow. A blouse or shirt that matches your skin tone is the most flattering. If you really want to wow them, then match your eye color, which will pull them right in for some direct eye contact. Although it may seem trite, candidates who use the right colors will be at a clear advantage.

The basics—hose, socks, shoes, and belt—should complement and not compete with the outfit. For men, the socks should match the pant color. For women, the hose should do the same; if the outfit is dark, wear black, blue, or gray hose. Pastel or bold colors are best complemented by neutral hose. The color of the shoes and belt should match and tastefully blend with the outfit's colors.

Accessories are the icing on the cake. If worn tastefully, they can complement an outfit and add sophistication and flare. On the other hand, gaudy jewelry or ill-matched accessories are distracting. The only acceptable piercings are in the ears. Sorry, guys, you don't get to wear any. And, ladies, limit yours to just two per ear. Jewelry should be understated yet sophisticated. Ties and scarves are a wonderful asset to express individuality as well as to capitalize on your best colors and good taste.

Hairstyle has a great effect on your appearance. For men, the length of hair is particularly important. You are trying to uphold the image of a clean-cut, well-groomed, board-certified obstetrician and gynecologist. This does not mean that you cannot have a beard or mustache, but if you do, it must be trimmed and orderly. For women, long hair pulled back by a barrette or in a pony tail may be seen as girlish and, therefore, unprofessional.

My final comments about appearance are trivial but help you to score points for style and attention to detail, such as using the term "leiomyomata" instead of fireballs. Fingernails should be clean and well manicured. If you choose to wear polish, it should be neutral and not ostentatious. Since you are a surgeon, your hands reflect your craft and are an indirect measure of how meticulous you are in the operating room.

Look carefully at your shoes. Make sure they are polished and not scuffed. Treat yourself to a professional shoe shine in the airport when you are en route to your exam. Likewise, your belt buckle should be polished, without areas of worn leather. Women should wear low heels—not high heels and not flats.

Don't underestimate the appearance of even your case list. At a minimum, staple the pages so that you don't accidentally trip and scatter it all over the floor. Better yet, organize it into a three-ringed binder, in which you can even put each page in a sleeve. The classiest touch of all is to have your copy professionally bound.

Appearance accounts for the majority of the first impression. The next factor, before you have even spoken one word, is the handshake. Because this is admittedly a stressful situation, you may well have cold and clammy hands. If they are like ice cubes, then stuff them into your pockets beforehand.

Your handshake should be firm but not bone-breaking. Women also should avoid a weak or limp-wristed handshake. You should look the examiner squarely in the eyes to project confidence and smile, albeit nervously.

The second most influential component of the first impression is voice quality. Because a first impression is made in only five seconds, the introduction is critical. Be aware of how anxiety and nervousness affect your speech. Practice the introduction until it is calm and projects confidence.

Consider standing out from the vast majority who will reflexively respond, "Nice to meet you" upon being introduced to the examiner. How about saying instead, "It's an honor to meet you"? A personal touch would be to add the examiner's name.

In conclusion, you cannot afford to underestimate the power of the first impression. Your case list has already evoked an initial mental image. The first five seconds of meeting you, however, leave a lasting impression. Attention to your image is merely another facet of testmanship. Strategizing how to enhance your image is as important as strategizing how to convey your knowledge. It is capitalizing on the age-old saying, "It's not what you say, but how you say it." You never get a second chance to make a great first impression.

# 10 Chapter

# The Oral Exam

Until 2000, *all* of the oral exams were conducted at the Westin Hotel in Chicago over *one week*, typically in early November. Since 2000, the exams are now given in Dallas, and they are spread out over *three months*. The candidates are divided into three groups and are examined over one week in each of three months: November, December, and January. The reason for this change is not clear. It certainly makes exam security a lot tougher, and major holidays—Thanksgiving and Christmas/Hanukah—are definitely ruined. Perhaps the board intends to use the same pool of examiners for all three months to promote standardization and consistency of exam conduct and thus afford a more accurate assessment of what constitutes pass/fail.

In the past, it was rumored that a minimum percentage of candidates was designated for failure. This change refutes that rumor, because the results of the exams are announced within two weeks. Obviously, the November results cannot be delayed until the January exams. Whatever the reasons for the change, it does not change your timeline for preparation. Once you know the date of your exam, back-plot the timeline for studying as recommended in Table 1 of Chapter 4: Getting Started. Given that the December and January dates coincide with the holidays, don't dillydally in making your airline reservations to Dallas.

## The Day Before

I strongly recommend you read Chapter 12: A Candidate's Journey both before and after you read the rest of this chapter to capture the emotions and stress experienced going into the exam. No matter how well you have prepared, you will be nervous …*very* nervous. You must understand and acknowledge how this anxiety affects your performance to truly be able to take the bull by the horns. To pretend that this is just another day at the office is foolhardy, naïve, and very risky.

I recommend that you arrive in Dallas at least one to two days before your exam. You need time to rally from unexpected travel delays. This is especially likely if your exam is in December or January, given the unpredictability of winter weather. Most of you will travel great distances and change time zones. You need time to recover.

Dallas is the home of the ABOG, and exams are conducted at the ABOG Test Center. The ABOG *Diplomate* reports that the test center has rooms designed specifically to accommodate the format of the oral exam. These accommodations include high-resolution computer screens with the capability of projecting Kodachromes and the case of the day. These screens are intended to "improve the image quality of the clinical condition under discussion." In the past, a projector for 35mm slides was set up in the hotel room, and images were projected onto the blank wall.

The ABOG *Diplomate* also reports that candidates will be housed in hotels within a six- to eight-block radius of the test center. The majority of the candidates stay at the Melrose Hotel simply because ABOG has contracted with them. Make your reservation right away, as the Melrose typically has no vacancy the week of the exam. In the past, candidates could stay at the Westin, where the exam was conducted and where the examiners also stayed. It was intimidating, to say the least, to meet the examiners in the restaurant or lounge or, worse yet, to see ashen-faced candidates stumble into the hotel lobby right after the test.

Regardless of your housing options, I recommend that you stay within a ten-minute walking distance of the Melrose. This recommendation is supported by the following example concerning a candidate who was staying about two hours away from Dallas. During the check-in, she realized that she had forgotten her case list. The exam was in one hour, and she did not have time to go back and get it. Of course, she had not memorized the case list and was helpless when asked by the examiners to defend patient #10.

Most of the examiners had made notes on their copies of her case list and were unwilling to share them. Needless to say, she was totally unnerved and failed. She attributed her failure to decompensating after simply forgetting her case list.

Regardless of where you stay, the night before the exam should be spent trying to relax. Do not attempt any last-minute cramming. If you feel compelled, skim over your case list. However, this is not the time for a night on the town. Try to get a good night's sleep. If you need a sleeping pill, make sure that you have tried it before to avoid a hangover for a morning exam. Set your unaltered case list and admission pass somewhere where you will all but trip over them the next morning. Remember, the case list you bring with you to the exam must be **identical** (except for the patient's initials) to the one submitted in August. It cannot include any notes, alterations, edits, etc.

## The Morning of the Exam

On the day of the exam, make sure that you eat. Although you are nervous, hypoglycemia will prevent you from performing at your peak. Take the time to primp. If you look good, then you will feel good. Dress conservatively and professionally. Use an anxiolytic if necessary, but make sure you have previously tested its side effects. If you have a good-luck charm, by all means tuck it in your pocket.

*Don't forget your case list*, your picture ID, and your admission pass. You may not bring pagers, cellular phones, computers, reference materials, nor briefcases to the registration, orientation or test center. If you are not staying within walking distance, then allow ample time for potential traffic delays.

On the day of your exam, report to the Melrose Hotel at your designated time. Each day there are two sessions, either morning or afternoon. Each session is preceded by breakfast or lunch.

There are typically 30 to 50 candidates per session. Following the meal, the ABOG executive director greets and welcomes you. He gives a friendly, uplifting, pep talk that reassures you that you are all smart and this is the most unimportant exam you will take.

Since this feels like your last day on earth, you are appropriately called up in pairs to receive your specific exam room number. You are requested to turn off and check in any pager, cell phone, computer, recorders, and any other electronic device. Thereafter, the presence of the above devices will be cause for immediate dismissal from the exam. You are allowed to bring a breast pump. Finally, you sign a declaration of "unrestricted privileges" and receive your photo ID badge. All the candidates are then shuttled about 10 or 15 minutes over the short distance from the Melrose Hotel to the ABOG Test Center.

Upon reaching the test center, you are greeted by other cordial and empathetic ABOG dignitaries. The first dignitary gives you an overview of the exam process by showing a five-minute vignette of the conduct of the exam. The next speaker, usually Director of Evaluation Dr. Larry C. Gilstrap III, tries to break the ice. He spends about 45 minutes with a humorous PowerPoint presentation, further expounding on what to and what not to expect. This includes dispelling myths, misperceptions, pass/fail statistics, and when to expect your results.

You then get to take a break and go to the bathroom. You definitely want to complete this necessity, as this is your last chance until after the test. Although you can theoretically go to the bathroom during the test, the clock does not stop. You will waste precious time, and you will want every single second to prove yourself. You are then instructed to go upstairs to the testing area.

Once there, you will report to your designated exam room. You remain in the same room while each pair of examiners rotate. The rooms are pleasant, well lighted, and have a window. You will sit on a rolling chair, on the window side of the desk, looking toward the door. On the left side of the desk is a flat-screen monitor. The corner of the screen has a clock with the real time. The examiners sit across from you at a tilt desk, attached to your desk, which contains their keyboard and papers. To your right is a pitcher of water. The examiners even pour you a glass at the beginning of the exam. The test begins at the sound of the computer chime.

## Exam Content

The exam is divided into three sections: obstetrics, gynecology, and office practice. Within each section, there are two categories: the case list and the case of the day.

Half of your exam is spent defending your case list, which reflects your mode of practice. The examiner can either refer to specific patients on your case list or use it as a springboard for other topics.

The other category is "structured cases" or "case of the day." The "case of the day," as discussed previously, is my term for the written narrative of a hypothetical patient management scenario. Each case of the day requires a standardized response. Although examiners may vary in their approach to each question, this format lends some objectivity to an otherwise predominantly subjective test.

## Exam Format

The exam lasts three hours, divided into three 60-minute blocks for each of the three sections: obstetrics, gynecology, and office practice. The 60-minute sessions can occur in any sequence. Half of each session is devoted to the case list and the other half to the case of the day. Effective in 2008, all candidates started with and completed all of the case of the day discussions before switching to the case list.

There are three pairs of examiners, one pair for each section. Typically, you are questioned by only one examiner at a time. The other observes and documents the conduct of the exam. The exam is also monitored by closed-circuit television with sound, but it is not recorded. One examiner will question you about the case of the day, and the other will question you about the case list. At the completion of each 60-minute segment. a chime sounds and the pair of examiners abruptly conclude, stand up, wish you well, and leave. Within one minute, the next pair of examiners will enter.

Although you are sitting for your general boards, traditionally the examiners are subspecialists. Usually the examiner is a specialist in maternal-fetal medicine for the obstetrics section, a reproductive endocrinologist for office practice, and an oncologist for the gynecologic section. Some of the examiners are generalists who can examine any of the three sections. Recently, a handful of urogynecologists have participated in the gynecologic section.

At any time during the exam, you are allowed to get up and go to the bathroom. This is not to your advantage as the clock does not stop. You also may make notes on the scratch pad, provided to you. Since you will be referring constantly to your case list, I recommend you organize it into a 3-ring binder with dividers between the 3 sections.

At the end of three hours, the exam is punctually concluded. You make a quick getaway downstairs. You must ride back on the shuttle to the Melrose, no exceptions. Don't cut your escape plans so tight that you miss your flight. Some head straight to the bar at the Melrose.

## Evaluation Criteria

The purpose of the exam is to assess your patient management acumen. The basis for patient management scenarios is derived from your case list, the cases of the day, and hypothetical patients. The ABOG gives these generic criteria for candidate evaluation:

1. Elicit data in an organized fashion.
2. Evaluate data and combinations of data.
3. Formulate a differential diagnosis.
4. Perform no harmful or unnecessary procedures.
5. Be familiar with diagnostic and therapeutic procedures.
   a. Indications
   b. Contraindications
   c. Complications
   d. Alternative procedures
6. Have an overall logical approach to patient care and treatment.

The examination is designed to evaluate your qualifications as a specialist or consultant to non-OB/GYN colleagues. Another goal of the test is to evaluate your behavior in independent practice. The emphasis is on patient management knowledge and skills.

The grading system is another highly-guarded secret. The best benchmark or standard to emulate is the ACOG standards. As long as your management is consistent with the ACOG guidelines in the *Compendium*, you will meet the passing criteria.

## Examiner Alerts

In 2000, the examiners were instructed to be kinder and gentler. Some do better than others in heeding this directive. Nonetheless, they are on a mission to "bring the cream to the top." Contrary to popular belief, their goal is to *pass* you. Unlike the written exam, the oral format strips control of the conduct of the exam from you and gives it to the examiner. An out-of-control rookie will undoubtedly crash and burn if not experienced and prepared.

The examiners write continuously. Do not misinterpret this as poor performance. They are legally required to document the conduct of the exam in case there are subsequent questions.

Examiners change topics abruptly once you have satisfactorily answered their question. They will even curtly interrupt you in the middle of a sentence to move on to the next topic. Don't misinterpret this as rudeness. Quite the contrary, they are doing you a favor in moving as quickly as possible. They have only thirty short minutes for each section. The more questions you answer right, the more you will dilute the wrong ones and obviously enhance your chances for passing.

Examiners will give you no feedback whatsoever. They will try to conceal facial, postural, or verbal gestures and to mask their approval or disapproval. In spite of this stiff environment, they usually are cordial and empathetic—with one exception.

Consistently there seems to be a "bad guy" in one of the three sections. ABOG formally denies the "good cop, bad cop" innuendos in the introductory slide show. I truly believe there is no designated hit man. However, think back to your residency. Name six faculty. I'll bet at least one was not known for his ooey-gooey sweet nature. It took you awhile to just accept him for who he was. You learned to look past this facet of his personality. You and his patients learned to be forgiving of his poor bedside manner, because he was a great doctor otherwise. Chances are that one of your six examiners is going to be less than kind, just because that's his nature.

Recently, the exam has not been as adversarial as it was reputed to be in the past. However, feedback from candidates since 2000 supports the continued existence of a not-so-friendly foe. It is usually quite obvious who it is. His job is to create a stressful environment to evaluate your decision-making ability under such conditions.

Because the bad guy cannot witness your performance in an actual life-threatening situation, he can only hope to simulate the same emotional response. Past tactics include openly displaying disagreement or dissatisfaction with your answers and impatience with your lack of quick decisions. He will even add emotion-provoking qualifiers to cloud your decisions—for example, making malpractice innuendoes or describing extreme social circumstances (e.g., emergency cesarean hysterectomy on a nulliparous patient).

Perhaps future examiners will be slapped on the hand for deviating from the kinder, gentler theme. I do know some examiners have been dismissed for this exact reason. However, it takes a bold, courageous, and mad-as-heck candidate to voice a complaint. But the ABOG is still in the process of change, and feedback from recent candidates confirms that not all examiners have jumped on the kinder, gentler bandwagon. Be prepared in case you don't get a convert.

Overall, try to stay focused on the issues and do not allow yourself to be forced into making hasty, careless decisions. Do not panic. Stay calm, cool, and collected. The more mock oral exams you take, the more skilled you become with interrogation under pressure.

## Exam Conduct

No doubt, your best preparation for an oral exam is to take mock oral exams. After all, repetition is the mother of learning, and practice makes perfect. Although you can never take too many, I recommend a *minimum* of three. The learning curve is definitely exponential.

Although you will discover many of the following tips on your own, prior knowledge of them before your first mock oral will save you from having to reinvent the wheel. Seeing is one thing, doing is another. Make sure that you get a chance to try these techniques during a few mock oral exams. Don't let your first time be the day of the exam.

Remember throughout the exam that "when in Rome, do as the Romans do." You are auditioning to join an elite club. *You* want to be one of *them*. Although you may not agree with their selection process, remember that you cannot change the system until you are in the system.

The exam is a humbling experience. Most candidates have invested one to two years in preparing for the exam. Your knowledge base of obstetrics and gynecology will be at its peak. Although the majority will pass, most candidates will feel like they failed when they leave the room.

You can't help but reflect on what went wrong. Remember that even after you successfully passed a topic, you will often be driven to the point where you must admit that you don't know. But that's their goal: to make sure that you know your limits and are humble enough to call for help. Just because you think that you didn't know the answer to many of the questions doesn't mean that you didn't pass the question and ultimately the exam. So forewarned is forearmed. If you walk out of the exam knowing you passed, that's a bonus.

The most valuable tip is to *answer only the question*. On the surface, this seems obvious. But most of us are used to a written exam, where the succinct answer is right there in black and white. You assume your verbal answer is as succinct but almost always feel the need to qualify your response further. The more you talk, the more you open other related topics. The examiner may have been perfectly satisfied with your answer, but your rambling opened a new topic. Since you brought it up, it's now fair game for discussion.

Listen carefully to the question. If you don't understand it, ask the examiner to repeat or clarify. Don't risk failing a question because of misinterpretation. If the examiner asks a close-ended question—"Did you do this or that?"—give a close-ended response: yes or no. The examiner who wants more information will ask. Try to answer open-ended questions as succinctly as possible. The exception is the topic on which you are well versed. Purposely lead the examiner into what you want to talk about. Undoubtedly, a few mock orals will help tremendously. Again, the bottom line is *answer the question*!

Accept responsibility for the patients on your case list regardless of who is at fault for dumping on you. The patient is on your case list; therefore, you own her. If it is important to convey injustice, say, "When I assumed her care, she was ..."

Avoid social, racial, or religious justification for a mode of practice unless appropriate. It would be inappropriate to justify your reason for induction of labor because a patient is of a stereotypic demanding religious sect. On the other hand, ordering certain labs because a patient is at risk for a disease because of his or her race or religion would be entirely appropriate.

Similarly, justify a planned breech of the standard of care. You may be precluded from following the norm of practice because of limitations within a group practice or hospital facilities. For example, you may not be able to offer methotrexate for non-surgical management of ectopic pregnancy because your elderly partners are uncomfortable with the drug. Perhaps you would like to offer laser vaporization of lower genital tract condylomata but are unable to do so because your rural hospital cannot afford a laser. Nonetheless, if you elect to violate the standard, simply acknowledge your understanding of the standard and support why you cannot adhere to it.

Speaking of standards, the ACOG standard of care is the standard by which you are judged. The ACOG *Educational and Technical Bulletins, Practice Bulletins and Patterns,* and *Committee Opinions* are the best references. They are packaged conveniently in the ACOG *Compendium*. Know them! Know what an OB/GYN consultant for non-OB/GYN practitioners would do—and don't go beyond the boundaries.

Settle the tug of war of "what I do vs. what I *should* do" ahead of time. For example, everyone has induced a patient for macrosomia, yet we all know that the ACOG evidence-based guidelines do not support this practice. So hopefully, if you are reading this before August 1, you can avoid this problem in the first place by simply listing it as an elective induction.

If you are now in case list defense mode, then acknowledge your understanding of the guidelines and shift the focus on how the patient was counseled.

The examiners are quite clever in pushing you to your limits. Don't say you would do something that normally you would not do. For example, if a complication of your breast cyst aspiration is a pneumothorax and the examiner asks you what is the next step, respond with, "Insertion of a chest tube." If the examiner wants to know the technique for placing a chest tube and you don't normally place chest tubes (as most of us do not), explain that you would consult your general surgeon and/or emergency department physician.

Once you have acknowledged your limitations, the examiner should back off. Sometimes, however, he or she may resort to below-the-belt tactics and make your consultant unavailable or ask what your consultant would do. This is probably a hint that the examiner expects you to know more. This is especially common in discussing intraoperative ureteral injuries. If you truly know what the consultant would do, answer the question. However, emphasize that you are not comfortable performing the procedure independently. If you do not know the answer, hold your ground and say that you will have to wait for the consultant.

Freely admit if you don't know. The examiner would rather hear an acknowledgment of your limitations than a foolhardy guess. If you guess, do so only if you are reasonably sure; otherwise, you will discredit yourself. They will try to trap you into going beyond your abilities, but don't fall for it. Admit if you don't know.

Don't change your answers. The golden rule for a written exam, "Never change your first answer," also applies to an oral exam. The examiners are skillful at manipulating you so that you end up second-guessing your answer. They often put words in your mouth. More cleverly, they will uncharacteristically grant you the opportunity to change your answer. Their encouragement and atypical empathy are just a facade. Their real agenda is to determine whether your decision making is certain and consistent.

Don't be overconfident. Arrogance is frowned upon and viewed in the same negative light as lack of confidence. This exam quickly puts you in your place. Rarely, there may be topics about which you are more knowledgeable than the examiner. Refrain from seizing the opportunity to lecture, teach, or argue. This is not the appropriate forum. Given that the examiners are judging you, this is not the time to embarrass or anger them.

Likewise, refrain from saying "the literature" says this or that. Then the examiner will ask you to specify exactly what you mean by "the literature"—

which journal, the authors, and so on. Don't fall into this trap. On the other hand, you may have indeed modeled a mode of practice after a specific article. It may be appropriate to reveal this, but be prepared to cite the specifics of the article. In addition, this will open the door for questions about how to review the literature critically, such as the power of the study and alpha and beta errors.

Perhaps the most difficult skill to master is to let a question go once you have answered it. Let bygones be bygones. Do not compromise the remaining questions by dwelling on the last one. Remember, you want to answer as many questions as possible, so the right answers will dilute the wrong ones. This is a skill that must be practiced, but once mastered, it will definitely be the ace up your sleeve.

## Points for Style

The following recommendations will win you points for style. These are subtleties that will raise your favorable impression a notch. They make up the gestalt, the hunch, the gut feeling the examiner has about you.

Again, listen carefully to the question. If you don't understand it, ask the examiner to repeat or clarify. Don't risk failing a question because of misinterpretation. Novice candidates will repeat the question with their answer. You shouldn't have to resort to this, as this is an age-old stall tactic used by those who are uncomfortable thinking before answering.

If you understand the question but need to ponder the answer, don't be afraid of silence. This is an enormous power play on your part. The ball is in your court. The examiner is powerless to move the exam on until you respond. This is not to be confused as a stall tactic. It is never to your advantage to slow the exam, as you want to answer as many questions as possible. However, being comfortable with silence is a rare trait that portrays a calm, cool, and collected candidate. It also assures you don't ramble nonsensically and open up a Pandora's box with unintended new ammunition for the examiner.

Try to maintain eye contact with the examiner. Don't you hate it when people won't look you in the eye when you're talking to them? What are they trying to hide? What are they afraid of? Don't they have confidence in what they're saying? Obviously, the same questions will be going through the examiner's mind, particularly when he compares you to the other candidates. Again, a few mock orals will fix this easily. I advise those who simply can't make eye contact to at least look directly at the examiner's nose.

Be aware of your posture and body language. Sit poised and natural. Remember, if you are not accustomed to wearing a suit, then you should wear it for at least one mock oral exam. Many of us have nervous tics that we are unaware of.

Express your thoughts verbally. After all, this is an oral exam. Do you talk with your hands? Some candidates especially succumb to using their hands to describe a procedure, such as how to deliver a breech vaginally or manage a shoulder dystocia. It's hysterical to watch a novice go through all the gestures and gyrations to demonstrate each maneuver. However, if you can articulate elegantly without supplementing with your hands, you will stand out hands down (pardon the pun) from the majority.

Be polite and respectful. I know this seems obvious, but I disagree with the advice to treat the examiner casually, like he is your partner or you are having a curbside consult. The oral board exam is anything but a casual affair; this is the biggest test of your career! The examiners are prestigious leaders in our field. I would address him/her respectfully as Doctor. Certainly, if you are comfortable, then also add ma'am or sir.

Accept responsibility for the patients on your case list. A common mistake in answering a question is to say "we," such as "we did this, then we did that." The exam is not a team effort—**you** are the only one sitting in the hot seat. The patient is on *your* case list; therefore she's *your* patient. Instead of "we," say "I."

Do not say *never* and *always*. These terms imply certainty in the inexact practice of medicine. Likewise, avoid the terms, *inadvertently, routinely, protocol*, or *that's how I was trained*. They imply resistance to change or comfort with the modus operandi, which is not the image of an up-to-date, board-certified obstetrician and gynecologist.

Chose your words carefully. The word *declines* vs. *refuses* is kinder and implies more neutral and informed counseling. For example, "The patient with a previous low transverse cesarean sections declined a trial of labor." However, you may want to say the patient refused a cesarean section for a non-reassuring fetal heart rate tracing to justify a mid-forceps delivery.

The examiners love when you humbly admit you made a mistake. Even better is to acknowledge, *I learned from this, and now I do this*. This is also an effective way to turn the tide in defending an obvious complication on your case list.

## The End of the Exam

A chime will signal the end of each hour-long segment. The examiners will abruptly conclude the exam and stand up to leave. You should stand up also to be respectful and shake their hand. *Smile, look them in the eye,* and *thank* them. Have the same firm handshake that you did when they first walked into the room. Remember to make a great lasting impression.

Whatever you do, do not request a repeat exam. I have heard this advice time and again from many different sources. According to the ABOG *Bulletin*, if a candidate feels that the exam was not conducted in a fair and unprejudiced manner, he or she may request a repeat exam within one hour of completion of the oral exam.

The examiners are typically experienced, with years of examining candidates. It is unlikely that your exam was really conducted unfairly and/or with prejudice. We will discuss how the results are tabulated in the next chapter. However, each pair of examiners independently determines your results. The examiners for one section have no idea who else is examining you. Use this to your advantage and recover if you bombed one section. Don't compromise the other two sections! Besides, statistically you have about an 85% chance of passing. Those odds are really in your favor.

If you think that you did poorly and that you will have a better chance the second time around, you have to wait until next year. The repeat exam is conducted by a different set of examiners who do not know that the candidate appealed.

The oral board exam is the climax of months of preparation. Admittedly, the bulk of your effort is building your knowledge base. The icing on the cake, however, is the persuasive articulation of your knowledge.

Few candidates can perform well and comfortably in an oral exam without practice. It's a shame to spend months on studying and not to devote a few hours to mock oral exams. Incorporating the above tips should give you the "razor's edge." With practice, you'll find that the oral exam format is actually easier to pass than the written exam.

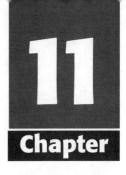

## Chapter

# Test Results

Historically, departing remarks were thought to contain clues as to whether or not you had passed the exam. "Have a nice flight" or "Enjoy the holidays" implied that you had passed. Believe me, there is no more guarantee in these remarks than there is in predicting the sex of a fetus by its heart rate. ABOG dispels this claim in the 45-minute introductory slide show.

The specific criteria for passing still remain a well-guarded secret. ABOG lists only generic criteria:

1. Elicit data in an organized fashion.

2. Evaluate data and combinations of data.

3. Formulate a differential diagnosis.

4. Perform no harmful or unnecessary procedures.

5. Be familiar with diagnostic and therapeutic procedures.

   a. Indications

   b. Contraindications

   c. Complications

   d. Alternative procedures

6. Have an overall logical approach to patient care and treatment.

The examination is designed to evaluate your qualifications as a specialist or consultant to non-OB/GYN colleagues. The goal of the test is also to evaluate your behavior in independent practice. The emphasis is on patient management knowledge and skills.

The best benchmark or standard of clinical care to emulate remains the ACOG standard. As long as your management is consistent with the ACOG guidelines in the *Compendium*, you will meet the passing criteria.

The ABOG *Diplomate* publishes the exam statistics annually. The pass rate for the oral board exam is higher than for the written board exam. The statistics are much in your favor. For the last decade, consistently from year to year, 85% of candidates pass their exam on their first attempt. Feedback from past board examiners provide some insight as to why the odds are so good. The computer matches you with your examiners based on where you trained and where you currently practice. You are provided this list on the morning of your exam to make sure there are no conflicts of interest.

Recall that you have three pairs of examiners. They will never put two junior examiners together. Each pair does not know who your other examiners are. For example, your obstetric examiners have no idea who is examining you on your office and gynecology sections. Within a pair, each examiner must grade you for the overall section. Even though an individual examiner will examine you on only half the test, either the case list or the case of the day, he records and observes the conduct of the exam by his co-examiner.

Typically a pair will examine three consecutive candidates. Remember how quickly the next pair of examiners enters upon the hourly chime? The examiners are playing musical chairs. Hopefully, the pair has the opportunity to converse at the end of each three-hour session and don't have to wait until the end of the day, after they've examined six candidates.

Each pair must be unanimous in their results. The options are pass, fail, or marginal. Each pair independently turn in their results.

The ABOG *Bulletin* states that the board of directors votes on each candidate based on the report of the examining team. Reportedly, a pass is awarded five points, a marginal three points, and a fail one point. You must score ten or more points in order to pass the exam, so do the math yourself. You will pass the exam with the following combinations: three pass; two pass and one fail or marginal; and one pass and two marginal.

The timing of the results suggests that the board votes at the end of the test week in each of the three months. The ABOG insists there is no preplanned pass/fail rate. I hope that the results are based simply on individual merit. ABOG is doing a better job in getting the results to you. In the past, it routinely took six weeks. Now you should have your results in two weeks.

Congratulations if you passed! Rest assured—but not for long. The clock starts ticking right away, and soon you must recertify. In 2008, they revamped the recertification process and even gave it a new name, Maintenance of Certification, or MOC.

Everyone must complete journal reading, with take-home tests every year. On the sixth year, you must take a written exam. Groan! I know you thought you were over that, but just like GERD, it has come back to haunt you. ABOG representatives have publicly acknowledged that the source for the written questions will most likely stem from the journal reading, so don't throw away those answer sheets!

Traditionally, the recertification written exam was a piece of cake— that is, if you are a generalist but bad news for you subspecialists. As you know, you have to maintain your generalist board certification. Everyone must take one of their two test books in general obstetrics and gynecology. If you are a generalist, then you get to choose your second book. The specialist must take the second book in his subspecialty.

In the unlikely event that you fail your oral board exam, you may repeat it twice—as long as you do so within six years of passing the written exam. After six years, you have to pass the written exam to start the cycle over. As awful as this seems, remember that in the past you had to repeat your *residency* to reset the clock.

## If You Fail...

So what if you fail the oral exam? What happens? Well, the easy answer is that you simply retake the exam. The hard answer is preparing you for the maelstrom of emotions that you will experience and need to process in order to be fit to take the exam again. If you are taking the test for the first time, read this chapter once and put it aside. If you fail the test, you must reread this again to understand that you are not alone and to learn from others' mistakes.

Back to the easy answer. You may retake the test the next go around. The problem is that it's a bit logistically problematic to pull it off that quickly. Even if you took your test during the first batch of exams, you won't get your results until around Thanksgiving. However, case list collections for the test the following year started July 1—or five months earlier. Of course, the situation is even worse if you did not take your exam until January. Talk about being behind the eight ball!

Of course, the shock and realization that you failed takes time to sink in. Everybody reacts differently. For those who react by taking the bull by the horns and regaining control, you can pull it off by recapturing the cases quickly. You certainly know what it takes, given you did it just recently. But for those of you immobilized by the dread of starting right back, then wait until the following July to start collecting.

Now for the hard answer. As with any major life stress, you will go through the Kübler-Ross stages of grief: denial, anger, acceptance, and resolution. Many of you will not be surprised that you failed, as you felt like you had already failed when you walked out of the test, especially as you began to ponder your answers. Actually, most candidates experience these same feelings, even when they did pass. Unfortunately, that letter from the executive director that starts, "Regretfully, I must inform you of your failure to pass the oral board exam..." validates your fear.

One of your toughest chores will be acknowledging to everyone that you failed. There is no escaping this embarrassing task because anyone who is in any way associated with you knows you've put your whole life on hold for this exam. Unfortunately, you have to inform your spouse, partners, office staff, friends, relatives, and the whole world. You feel like there's a billboard in front of your house or office or your forehead is branded with: "I failed my oral board exam."

Although you are humiliated and embarrassed, life quickly moves on for others. Think about it: When you hear a rumor or gossip, how long do you linger on it? Probably only for as long as it took to hear it, right? Do you know any of your colleagues that failed their boards? Do you no longer refer patients to them? Have you ever heard of patients not coming or transferring their care for this reason? The answer is **no**! Although this will leave a scar on you, it will not leave even a scratch on anyone else. Life will move on, and time softens the blow. You'll know when you're ready to face it again. You must get back in the saddle. Your first task is to figure out, objectively and without emotion, why you failed.

So **why** did you fail? The most common reason cited in that generic letter is "failure to defend your case list." Most admit they simply failed to prepare adequately. The more uncommon reasons are stage fright or exam anxiety or the candidate had no idea. Try to figure out why you failed so you can better prepare yourself next time. Most will acknowledge the

"Lessons Learned" noted in Chapter 13. Your strategy next time is simple. You need to prepare academically and psychologically.

Many candidates find the harder of the two is the psychological preparation. Clearly, our own training in counseling for depression and anxiety is dismal. So why do you feel you are now an authority to get yourself out of this hole? You wouldn't advise your patient to go it alone, so neither should you.

You will heal emotionally far quicker is you seek a counselor—a member of the clergy, a psychologist, or a psychiatrist. It is well known that many world-class athletes will seek the support of a sports psychologist. You're no different. He will help you "mind your mind" and help to restore balance.

This time around, keep all the balls in the air, instead of just one. Do not put life on hold. It didn't work before and chances are it won't again. Budget for and embrace personal and family time. A step away from studying rejuvenates the soul and makes you far more effective when you do study.

This time, take the time to develop a study plan as discussed in Chapter 8. Tackle your case list with the vigor and intensity that only a wizened veteran possesses. But this time you **must** take mock orals. Almost all who failed admitted they neglected this critical step. Why? Because they viewed this as an acknowledgement of their weakness rather than as a learning tool. What initially is viewed as a confidence shaker quickly becomes a confidence booster. I promise this is the key to your success next time.

When you retake the exam, the examiners do **not** know that you failed before. You really are at an advantage because now you do know what to expect. Make sure you heed that old proverb, "Trick me once, shame on you; trick me twice, shame on me." Finally, you will learn and grow from this, for "that which does not kill us will make us stronger."

# 12
## Chapter

# A Candidate's Journey

I have been mentoring candidates preparing for their board exams for nearly twenty years. Yet it seems like only yesterday when I went through that miserable process myself. Although the blood, sweat, and tears have long dried, I wanted to capture those emotions to help others know what to expect, as forewarned is forearmed.

Everyone's journey is unique, yet we share that same quest to put FACOG behind our beloved MD. I met KJ at our April review course. She was preparing for her oral exams the following fall. I am always impressed with those who have the foresight to be so proactive, as most will delay attending the review course until the fall of the exam. Coincidentally, KJ and I ran into each other at the airport after the course. I knew she was from my state, but discovered she actually practiced only about an hour from me; thus, we were on the same flight. Naturally, we began to chat.

I applauded her for being ahead in the game. She confessed that actually she was not preparing for the oral exam at all, but rather for the written boards *again*. She had failed her written exam and was devastated. "I had *never* failed anything in my life. I was crushed, humiliated, and demoralized. You are actually only the second person I've told. Only my husband knows. I couldn't even tell the rest of my family, friends, nor even my partner."

We physicians are so darn tough on ourselves. But it's true, we don't accept defeat well. Heck, we're devastated if we get a B, but to *fail*? I truly believe that there is no way anyone can make it through four years of college, four years of medical school, and four years of residency if he weren't smart. Can you still practice OB/GYN without being board certified? Yes. But it's not the same without that FACOG behind and lifting up that MD. You know it, I know it, and our colleagues know it. Our patients, on the other hand, only understand the MD part.

So this failure, this defeat is a crushing blow. However, I have yet to meet a colleague who hasn't acknowledged that picking herself up, and facing and overcoming that defeat was one of the most profound growing experiences of her lifetime. KJ was no exception.

We reflected on the past. It turns out she had poorly prepared the first time. She admitted her strength was always as a clinician, not an academician. Her residency did not provide financial, scheduling, academic, or emotional support. She used her vacation time to attend a review course, but her 80- to 100-hour work week did not permit the necessary time to embrace the material.

Well, you usually get out of it what you put into it. Although she was now very busy in private practice, job #1 was to pass her boards. This time she put her all into it. She passed her written board exam on her second attempt.

She was determined to not make the same mistake twice. Trick me once, shame on you; trick me twice, shame on me. As soon as KJ called me with the good news, I asked her to keep a journal of her journey.

She has attacked preparing for her oral exams with zeal. Although now, you might argue, she's not the typical candidate since she has some baggage, she nonetheless is undertaking this project for the first time. Let's take a peek into her diary.

**July 1**. "I feel much better about the written exam this time. I really think I did my best. If I failed, it will be hard to figure out what to do differently, but until I know my results, I'm going to proceed full steam ahead. I dug out my ABC (America's OB/GYN Board Review Course) notes. I'm really glad I went to those sessions on case list construction. I didn't so much understand it then, but it was clear that the case list is the biggest player in the exam, and you want to get it right the first time. I recall a lot of complaints about the ABOG software, so I'm going to order the ExamPro software today."

Starting on day 1 of case list collections, KJ started two files: one for gynecology and the other for obstetrics. The GYN file contained the admitting history and physical, operative note, discharge summary, pathology report, and office notes for each patient she operated on. The OB file contained the office prenatal record, the admitting history and physical, delivery/operative notes, discharge summary, and postpartum visit.

Admittedly, this approach is definitely exploding out of the starting blocks. Because you can't formally apply for the oral exam until November, many will naively not start any work on their case list until then. This is a big mistake, as they are already five months behind. I think KJ is right on, and would strongly recommend you model her record keeping approach.

Also, many erroneously but innocently assume you must use the ABOG software. This is not true. ABOG mandates only that your list must exactly duplicate their headings. The ABOG software, although much improved over the years, still has some bugs. There are a number of commercial software products that are available too.

**August 7.** "I got my letter from ABOG today. I was afraid to open it. I held it up to the light. I could see the word "Congratulations," so I tore it open. **I passed! Thank you, God!** I am so glad that's behind me. Life is good. Now I'm pumped up and am going to start entering my cases today."

Good news is a great motivator. I think it is reasonable to wait until you for sure know you passed your written boards before you begin entering your cases. This applies, of course, only for those who choose to take their oral boards immediately after their written boards. If you choose to take a break the year after your written board exam, then there is no excuse to delay. You should have your case list software in hand and start entering cases in July.

**September.** "I am entering my cases weekly. I have the hang of it now. I don't think this artificial intelligence with the ExamPro software is as helpful as I thought it would be. Most of the prompts are self-explanatory. Funny how you don't have any control about the type of cases. I find with every patient I see, I wonder how it's going to play out on my case list."

**October.** " I got my passport pictures taken today for my application. I told Paul [her husband] I felt like I was getting my mug shot taken for prison. Case list collections going well. I find it's easier to just enter them at the end of the day. I know I'm probably adding way too much information, but I figure I can always delete extraneous information later."

**November.** "Well, I sent my application in today. It felt good to formally get the ball rolling. I can't believe it's so expensive to just apply. I'm going to have to deal out another $900 just for the examination fee. Oh well, it sure beats the alternative."

**January 6.** " I met with Dr. Das today, just to make sure I'm on track, since I'm at the halfway mark. I figure it will be easier to fix problems now. She made me look at the list in a way I never even thought of: that is, from the *examiner's* perspective. Gee, why didn't I think of that? It makes sense. It's far more logical to word the cases *before submission* to strategically control the questions that **I** want **them** to ask me.

"She also showed me her case list library. These are binders filled with case lists. She very quickly convinced me how the *physical appearance* of a case list makes a huge impression. When you have the luxury to look at a big stack of case lists, I realized the outstanding ones were obvious within seconds. Of course, my only perspective until then was my own.

"She showed me some of her favorites; these were obviously customized. She told me that one of them was created by the teenage son of a candidate. Several others she claimed were drafted in the evenings of the review course. Could it really be *that easy*? I've got 6 months left. I don't want to have one of those cookie cutter case lists. I want to stand out. I'm going to create her new favorite."

Note that KJ deliberately did not start with the ABOG case list software. However, she discovered the commercial software did not meet her expectations either. Sometimes you have to appreciate what you don't like in order to help you better define what you do want. She has plenty of time to transition to a different program.

**January 12.** "I have been working with Debbie (ABC's operations manager and a "computer genius" according to Dr. Das) by e-mail, but today we met. I showed her how I created my custom case list with Microsoft Word using tables. She had recommended Excel spreadsheets, but she likes my idea. Admittedly, my timing for this project was lousy, since I upgraded to Vista. It's difficult to create a case list, learn about something in Microsoft that I have never used before, *and* figure out the new Vista all at once. This would be horrible if it was June and the deadline was quickly approaching!"

Amen to the not putting if off until the end! KJ had the luxury to work with Debbie Patrick. Obviously, she was able to meet with her since she was geographically close. In this day and age, however, you can easily obtain a consult by teleconference, videoconference, e-mail, etc. There are also case list construction workshops that are available starting in the later winter or early spring. It is interesting that KJ, through experimentation on her own, was able to present a new way, even to a seasoned veteran.

**February.** "My spiffy new case list is polished and much better organized. Reentering the cases was very good because it made me rethink the cases. I threw out details that were not important and added ones that I missed previously. Dr. Das will not have to use much of that red ink next time, that I'm sure!"

**March.** "Began to collect my office cases. I gave Kristie [her medical assistant] a list of the office practice categories. She is really taking it to heart. She'll whisper in my ear, 'This would be a good one for your case list'".

**April.** "Pulled out my ABC case list construction notes and reread Dr. Das's book. I'm starting to shift cases and reword [the notes], trying to put some strategy. Starting to pull references for topics."

By this time, you get routed into a habit. It's good to revisit the whole issue, as now you are able to appreciate hints and tips that you glossed over earlier. This is definitely a fluid process. If you haven't already, this is a good time to invest in a case list construction workshop.

**May 20.** "Met with Dr. Das ,and we reviewed my OB and office case list. Does this lady ever run out of red ink??! Discovered I have bullet toxicity (no, not the one from the gun, but after that session, doesn't sound like a bad alternative). Learned bullets for the OB are a completely different organizational tool than for the GYN case list. Decided to put that project on hold until after Army Reserve Annual Training. I'll prioritize getting the office collections done and be up to date on OB and GYN collections."

Ideally, you need to have your case list reviewed for construction tips about this time. This gives you plenty of time to deliberately word and place cases exactly to meet your strategic objective.

**June.** "Met one last time with Dr. Das. My case list is just about ready to go. There is very little red ink this time. I am having some formatting challenges, but for the most part I am satisfied with the outcome. I feel sorry for those who waited until the last minute and are fighting with their office staff and medical records for data. I am glad I started this process early. And I'm glad I had a mentor in this process. I can't imagine doing it alone."

**July 3.** "Received letter from ABOG that my application has been accepted. I also was surprised they said my exam is in January. Gosh, they haven't even received my case list, yet I already have my exam date… or at least the month of my exam. I have mixed emotions. I wish it was in November; then I would be done with it earlier, but then again, it will give me more time to prepare."

**July.** "I'm pleased with my second draft. It really paid off to work so hard earlier, because it's so easy to make the changes now. It's going to be weird not working on this anymore. I feel like it's part of my daily routine. I'm doing fine on time."

**July 23.** "Sent my case list—**taking no** chances of UPS losing it. I have my tracking number and sent it signature request receipt so ABOG has to verify they received it. Boy, do I feel like a huge weight has been lifted off my shoulders. I have no regrets with how I constructed that list."

**August, September.** "Since my exam is not until January, I've gone fishin'. I'm going to play, have fun, and *not* think about the boards or that case list at all."

June and July is all consuming with finishing the case list. It's a good idea to take a break. If your exam is in November, then you can't step away for as long as those whose exam is in January.

**October 21.** "I went to ABC's Oral Exam Workshop … talk about an eye opener. We were paired up and reviewed each other's case list. You could tell some were just thrown together with little thought. Some people left themselves wide open for questions about topics that no one wants to discuss. Some lists were boring with "DUB" over and over again and the same management every time. Some people did not follow directions about the number of cases on the office list (40) or about making the lists HIPAA compliant. I felt very good about my case list and now know that it was well worth the time and effort that I put into it.

"On the other hand, I need to study! During the workshop, I volunteered to be in the hot seat, and the other candidates quizzed me. I could answer some of their questions, but I could tell that most of them had been studying while I was goofing off in August and September. No more break for me! Now I'm ready to focus during the Review Course for the next five days."

**October 22-26.** "I attended the ABC Board Review Course. During that time, I made a study plan. Some of the topics I knew well, but it seems like I learned new things even during those lectures. Throughout the course, I made a list of one-liners, things I had always meant to learn/memorize but never seemed to have the time, to study later. I highlighted some things in the syllabus during the lectures, but because my focus is more clinical this time, I spent more time *listening* rather than just writing down every word. The speakers were excellent so I actually enjoyed listening too. I especially liked how exam focused they were, so it helps me focus my studying.

"We "oral exam takers" gave each other mock oral exams about the lectures during the breaks. One of my favorite parts about the course was meeting people like me who were as panicked. We met in the evenings to study too, because a few had to sit for their boards in less than two weeks. I'm glad that's not me, but on the other hand, I wish it was."

**November 7.** "Met with Dr. Das to just strategize what to do from now until my exam. I told her I'm going to take a few weeks off over the holidays and really focus on studying without my pager or patient responsibilities. Paul and I are going back home and travel for two weeks over Christmas. We get back on Sunday, January 4. I have explained to Paul that I won't be able to socialize because I have to study. Dr. Das has insisted that I spend some quality time with family without guilt about not studying. It is very hard to find balance. Still haven't heard the exact date of my exam, but worse case scenario, if it's the Monday, then I'll have eight days left. Dr. Das suggested we schedule a mock oral in December before I leave and then immediately upon my return. Damn, now I'm starting to get nervous. Maybe I shouldn't have blown off studying in August and September. It's too late to cancel my trip and Paul would kill me. Okay, not to panic. I can do this.

"I am studying for about two hours a day and 6-8 hours on the weekends. I am actually enjoying it quite a bit since this is about my patients. Previous studying has been to answer a specific question. This time I am studying to have a discussion about a patient. This is what I do every day when someone "curbsides" me about a patient or when I discuss patients with colleagues. In my day-to-day conversations with my partners I am practicing for my oral boards."

**December 7.** "Took the day off yesterday to spend time with family, and today I am studying. Meeting with MFM for mock oral Dec 9 after work. I am going to review my OB notes and case list before the meeting so I can be prepared. This will be my first mock oral so I don't really know how I am going to do, but I'm not too nervous because I discuss patients with her pretty regularly."

**December 8.** "Spoke with local REI, and he has agreed to meet with me in January. Has even offered to buy dinner because he knows what I'm going through. I got my letter with the date for my oral exam. Last day, last session. I guess I get more time to prepare than almost everyone else taking the boards. I'm not sure if this is good or bad. More time to worry too.

"I called the local hotels for reservations but a lot of them are sold out. A couple people have advised me not to stay at the Melrose because it is pretty noisy and difficult to sleep. I don't think I'll be sleeping much at that point anyway, but I'll take their advice. Made reservations to arrive on Jan 14 for my Jan 16 exam. That should give me a little quiet time away from my beeper, office and family responsibilities."

**December 10.** "I met with the MFM for a case list review and mock oral last night. She gave me some really good pointers. She advised me to always repeat the question because it gives time to think and to only answer the question asked. This makes sense to me. She pulled some topics out of my case list that she is pretty sure the examiners will ask. She didn't really ask me any questions, and I didn't ask her to because I was afraid that I wouldn't know the answers. Ugh! Isn't that why I asked for this meeting? Isn't it better to be miserable now so that I won't be as miserable later????"

You need to give your mock oral examiner guidance on how to conduct the session if they have no experience. Refer back to Chapter 8 for that list. Although volume is helpful, the more mock oral exams, the better; it's even more helpful if you get a quality exam. Remember *perfect practice* makes perfect.

**December 16.** "*&^**!#! Met with Dr. Das last night for mock orals. **Miserable!!!** She really knows how to find the little things that I don't know, and magnify them. Who cares about "mechanism of action"? I know it works and how to use it. I need to go home and hi-light [sic] all the drugs on my case list and memorize the MOAs so the examiners won't be able to make me as miserable as she has. I guess I don't have much of a poker face because she could tell every time the questions she asked were out of my comfort zone. I need to learn to relax and not tense up and start stuttering when I don't know the answer to a question right away. I will be sooooo happy when this whole process is over! I know how to take care of patients, and this is very frustrating!

"I still haven't done any Christmas shopping, sent any cards or attended a party. It seems like all I do is study and work. I can't wait for my vacation next week. I know I can get some real studying done if I get out of town and away from my pager."

**December 26.** "Landed in Frankfurt, Germany, today. I reviewed all of the GYN sections of my notes in the airport and on the flight. I got a lecture from Paul about ruining the trip by studying too much, but we discussed this before we made the reservation. I have promised to spend some free time with him, but my goal is to focus on studying for the boards."

**December 27.** "It was a great day today strolling from one café to another. Coffee and amenorrhea...Hot chocolate and the new Pap guidelines...chocolate and postpartum hemorrhage... I hope I can still fit into my suit when I get home."

Regardless of when your exam is, at least one, if not both, of your holidays are ruined. By this time, studying and the looming exam are heavy on your mind. Remember to at least budget time off and stick to it! You will feel less guilty, your family will be appreciative, and your studying will be more focused.

**December 30.** "Okay, now I am stressing out. I should have finished the first review of all the notes by now. I only have 3 weeks to go, and we are heading to see family today. How am I going to get everything memorized in time? Maybe I should have stayed home."

You will always feel like you can study more. There will always be some items left over on your study list.

**January 1.** "I haven't studied in 2 days. I keep thinking about how Dr. Das said to spend some quality time away from my studies and enjoy my family. I needed a break, but now I'm ready to buckle down again. How would I possibly do this if I had kids? My friends set up a little office for me complete with drinks, snacks, and Internet. I feel guilty studying instead of visiting, but we told everyone about my "important test" before we made the reservations. Everyone is wishing me luck and praying for me to pass. How miserable is it going to be if I don't pass? This pressure is all consuming. Everyone at the hospital knows I'm sitting. Everyone at my office knows. What if I don't pass?  How will I face everyone? "

**January 7.** "Back to the good old USA. I am back on track and on schedule. I met with my local REI for a mock oral on my office case list. We went one case at a time, and he quizzed me for 3 hours. At 3 different times he told me I was going to pass. Yeah! My studying is paying off. This was a little too easy. I hope the examiners are as reasonable as he was."

**January 8.** "Another mock oral and round robin with Dr. Das. I don't know how she does it, but she can find the little things that you thought you knew but obviously didn't know well enough. She busted me again on those stupid MOAs. This no feedback thing is tough. How do you know if you are answering the questions correctly? It's no wonder when most people leave the exam they think they've failed. I sure hope I don't feel that way. Too many people are counting on me to pass."

**January 13.** "I think I'm gonna throw up! My husband said goodbye and good luck to me this morning, and could feel the tears welling up.

What if I don't pass? I don't want to have that conversation, "I know you did your best...Those stupid people don't know anything...You are the best doctor I know..." What if I start crying when the examiner asks me something I don't know? What if I just sit there and can't think? What if I forget the mechanism of action of methotrexate? Can they fail you for that? What if I don't pass? How humiliating!

"This pressure is all consuming and not worth it! I wonder if there is someone else as stressed out about this stupid process as I am. Maybe I'm crazy. I know I must have studied enough to pass, but what if the examiners can find my weaknesses as easily as Dr. Das can? I had my colleagues quiz me, and I knew almost all of the answers to their questions. My studying has definitely made me more confident with them. I know a lot. I know enough to pass. **I will pass!!!**

**January 13.** "My flight leaves at 7AM, so I'm staying at a hotel by the Asheville airport. Dr. Das came for one last hoorah session. I was hoping to bribe her with desert [sic], as I've figured out she usually softens with this tactic. She just got back from Dallas last night giving ABC's mock oral exams just before the test. She's been in the office all day, then a dinner meeting and unfortunate for me, already had desert [sic]. She looked tired, but seemed to really perk up at the thought of torturing me with my final mock oral.

"Reviewed vaginal breech, TVT vs. TOT and more. I know a lot more now than I did the last time we got together. However, she managed to pull out a drug that wasn't even on my case list. That's simply not fair. I had told her after our last encounter that I was going to learn all the MOAs for each drug on my case list, so she demanded to quiz me on my drug cards. She tried to bore right through me, but I stood my ground. After going through half the deck, she conceded and retreated, and acknowledged I knew them well. **Hah!!** One for **me**, and a big fat zero for Das. I'm ready, let me at 'em.

"She told me that I deserve to pass. I know I must deserve to pass but I'm not perfect and neither is my knowledge base. I have a little more to study over the next few days but she says it's too late to learn and I think she's right. I need to relax. I can't remember if I know how to do that."

The week of the exam is the toughest. What's done is done. There's nothing more to do. You can't possibly learn anything more, and that reality just hits you squarely in your face. Now you have to accept that you have no more control...and that's depressing and terrifying. There is no turning back. You've waited so long for this week, yet it is suddenly here. You must get yourself psyched up. **Only** *positive* thoughts: "**I will pass**. I think I can. No, I **know** I can. Yay me!!"

**January 14.** "Arrived in Dallas without a hitch. There's a blizzard in Chicago. I hope those people gave themselves a little buffer. I doubt ABOG will be too sympathetic about acts of nature. I'm sure they would be happy to let those folk come back next year no charge.

"I am staying at a Marriott Hotel because I heard the Melrose was too noisy to study [in]. I need time away from everything and time to breathe, to focus and to figure out how not to freeze when the questions start. I think I am hypercritical of myself because I know the pain of failure. I don't want that to happen again. This is a very emotional time for me, and I can't freak myself out thinking about it too much. I made reservations for a massage and facial tomorrow. Reviewed a few things before bed, but nothing is sticking in my brain anymore."

It's a good idea to arrive one or two days before. The winter weather is unpredictable, and it's risky to have no wiggle room in case of delays. If you will have a time zone change, then you need time to acclimate. There are pros and cons at staying at the Melrose, which is where you meet the day of the test. Some want to be in that environment and own it! Others want to avoid it like the plague. What is your strategy? Get a good night's sleep tonight, but the night before your exam will be restless."

**January 15, DAY BEFORE.** "Aaaaahhh! Leisurely breakfast…massage with Gabriel, facial with Leslie…Now I'm ready. One more quick look at my notes because I feel obligated. I wonder what the other applicants are doing now. Probably cramming. 24 hours from now and it will all be over. I won't put myself through this process again. Too much pressure! I hope I pass. I hope I can sleep tonight. I'm glad I'm not staying at the noisy Melrose."

Try to relax. Do whatever it takes. Treat yourself. You deserve it. No studying.

**January 16, EXAM DAY 0300 (3am).** "Test day. Can't sleep. The bed is comfortable and the room is quiet, but I'm getting excited. I'm ready. I know I'm ready. I wish I were in the morning group. I should try to get some more sleep or I'll be feeling my usual sleepiness in the afternoon. I definitely won't be having coffee with lunch because we won't get a bathroom break for 3 hours. I'm a little nervous about that. Even if I have to go, I'll hold it so the wrong answers I give will count for less. Hmmm…If I am doing well and they ask something I don't know should I then ask for a bathroom break?? I'm over-thinking again. I'm going back to bed."

**January 16, EXAM DAY 1000 (10:00am).** "Okay, so I've said my final goodbyes to everyone, and I have prayers and brainwaves coming from every direction, and I'm freaking out. I have no good reason to freak out, and I'm freaking out. I am so afraid of failure it hurts. Dr. Das just sent a text message: "Remember, just 70%." I love this woman. She absolutely knows what to say to ease your mind. I don't have to be perfect. Just 70%. Time to get dressed and stop crying. I'm such a baby. If my referring docs could only see me now!"

**January 16, EXAM DAY 1030 (10:30am).** "I look sharp! This suit is great. The shoes are good. My hair is just right. I'm gonna knock 'em dead!!! Case list, ID, no cell phone. I'm outta here. The next time I see this room I'll be finished with the boards!"

**January 16, EXAM DAY 1700 (5pm).** "It was definitely an exhausting day. I really felt like they tried to make it even more dramatic than it needed to be with all of the procedural stuff. They give you a time to be at the conference room at the hotel, and then have you all sit in this room with a bunch of stressed people in suits waiting until the specified time. Then instead of registering you as you came in, they call you up front to register in groups of two. It really just dragged the whole process and made everyone even more nervous!

"I'm 90% sure I passed, but I'm 100% done. Yahoo!!! That wasn't too bad. I heard stories from others that they had really tough examiners, but mine were reasonable. It was tough when they grabbed on to something I wasn't sure about, but that's my fault.

"The things I didn't know were things I would have never considered studying (like what percentage of Synthroid crosses the placenta?) or were things I had reviewed but just forgot at the moment. There were a lot of differential diagnosis questions, especially in the case of the day questions. I really thought the case list questions were straightforward and easy— because I knew my case list well. I thought that was easier than the case of the days simply because I knew what to expect and was more prepared for those questions.

"I'm a good doctor. I am a good obstetrician and gynecologist. I may not know it all, but I know how to find the answers when I need them. If I don't pass this test, I don't know what else I could possibly do to better prepare. I passed. I'm sure of it. But I don't want to jinx it, so I'll say 90%. Time to celebrate being done!!!!

**January 17, Day After.** "Woke up with a headache this morning. I am trying not to think about the test too much, but I keep thinking of things I may have answered incorrectly. They asked about a 40-weeker with a precipitous delivery of an 1800g baby. All I could think of was the ddx for IUGR, and we talked about that for a while. I think they really wanted to know about resuscitation, but I didn't figure that out until about 4am. Oh jeez! This is torture!"

**January 21.** "I dreamed last night that I opened the envelope and it said "We are sorry to inform you…" I woke up **very** relieved that it was only a dream. I have been trying to keep busy so I don't have time to think about it, but the wait is killing me."

**January 22.** "I got a call from Dr. Das this afternoon that a guy in Virginia got his scores today. Now I'm afraid to go home and check the mail. I won't let Paul check because I don't want him to have to think of a way to let me down gently. I was 90% sure I passed, but now I'm only 70% sure. Part of me wants to hurry home, but part of me hopes that I don't get the letter today. If it doesn't come I can still be 70% sure I passed instead of 0%."

**January 23, 11:00am.** "No mail yesterday. I saw patients this morning and made my office manager cancel my afternoon meeting with my accountant. If I fail, I won't be able to pay attention, and if I pass I won't be able to pay attention. My sister says the mailman comes between 11:30 and 11:45am while I'm at work. She knows this because she waits for him often. She even knows his name and all about his children. Maybe I should ask her to put in a good word for me. Everyone in the office knows I'm going home to check the mail. If I fail I am not going to get out of bed this weekend, and I might stay in bed next week too. I will be "certified nuts" if not board certified. UGGGhhhh….this waiting is awful!"

**January 23, 11:45am** "Yahoo!!!!!! I passed!!!!!!!! OMG I can't believe it!!! Yes I can!!!!! I knew I would pass!!!!!!!!** I carried the envelope from the mailbox into the kitchen because I was afraid to see what was inside. I opened it with Paul and I saw the word "Congratulations!" That's all it took to make me start sobbing like a baby. Paul kept saying, "No, it's okay, **you passed**!!!" I had no idea what the rest of the letter said, but the first word was, "Congratulations!" You know me… I started thinking… I wonder if it says, "Congratulations… You failed and get to start the whole wonderful process over again!" I made Paul read the whole letter to me, but I didn't really hear what he was saying after the first few lines. I started calling and texting everyone I know, starting with Dr Das. No one knows how much this test meant to me more than her. It felt so good to have the people that mean so much to me texting back their congratulations. One of my friends even shouted out the good news to everyone in the hospital cafeteria! Another asked if she could put it on **her** Facebook page because she was so proud of me."

*Afterthoughts:* "If I had it to do all over again (**which I don't!!!**) I would do everything the same way. I am very lucky to have failed my written boards the first time. That might sound crazy, but I didn't know what I didn't know. What I mean is failing made me truly embrace the learning process.

"In residency I was groomed to believe that I knew more than my peers because of our powerhouse program. That was not true. I am a very good and capable surgeon, but my academic skills were lacking because no one expressed to me the importance of academics. Sure, I learned all about specialized research and how to care for the zebras, but I missed out on a lot of the basics. Like most of us, I had never failed anything before in my life. It was devastating to get the letter telling me I was a failure at what I had just spent 120 hrs a week for the last four years doing. It didn't really say I was a failure, but that's what it felt like. I was devastated and humiliated, and I told **no one** except for my husband and later Dr. Das.

"After I picked myself up, I vowed to study like I was in medical school again, and I did. I took Dr. Das's ABC course and memorized everything in the huge binder. I could even quote the ACOG *Compendium*. I passed my written board exam on the second try, and I passed as a much better physician, not only a good clinician but a good academician.

"I started this journal just after I passed the written exam, and I studied for another 18 months. This time I studied while I cared for my patients. Because the oral exam is all about how you function as you care for your patients, I actually enjoyed the process. There was a lot of stress for me because of the previous failure and all the emotions that that created, but I think that has made passing the oral exam that much sweeter.

"You won't find a mentor more passionate about her job than Dr. Das. She went far above and beyond my expectations because she genuinely cares. I think she feels responsible for making sure all of her protégés succeed, and this is what makes her stand out among her peers. If you think you can't do it, call her. If you need to relearn the basics, sign up for an ABC course. Go early in the year to give yourself time to study. Get help with case list construction so you have a better chance of discussing topics **you** want to discuss rather than those you don't. Put yourself through mock orals with anyone who will talk to you, and if you can, make an early reservation to have Dr. Das or one of her ABC staff **torture** you too. There was almost nothing that the examiners asked me that I hadn't heard before either at the ABC course or one-on-one with Dr. Das.

"Good Luck!"

—KJ, MD, FACOG

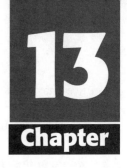

## Chapter

# Lessons Learned

After the exam is over and the dust has settled (or, perhaps more appropriately, after the blood, sweat, and tears have dried), I have asked candidates, "If you had to do it all over again, what would you do differently?" Below are the most frequent responses.

1. **Start collecting my case list earlier and updating it more frequently (regularly).**

   *Recommendation:* Ideally, you should start the process on July 1. Begin collecting and entering your gynecologic cases *after every surgery* and your obstetric cases *after every delivery*. Put some blank case list forms in your locker on Labor and Delivery, in your office and your briefcase. Better yet, put a form in the patient's office chart when you head over to surgery, and fill it out in the operating room after you dictate the procedure. Match these rough drafts with the accompanying history and physical, operative or delivery note, and discharge summary.

   If you cannot update your case list after every surgery or delivery, then do so *at least weekly*. If you procrastinate longer than two weeks, then you will have lost recall of precious details. In the long term, you will waste more time and experience more frustration in trying to capture lost dates and details.

   For the office case list collection, I recommend that you keep a list of the 40 categories on your desk starting in August. Over the next few months, simply jot down the patient's name and diagnosis when they fit a particular category. Once you have four names in a category, cease further collection. Every two to three months, pull the corresponding office chart and develop a rough draft case list for each one. At the five- to six-month mark, begin an earnest search for those hard-to-find categories. In May, select your final 40 patients.

### 2. I would not use the ABOG computer program for case list collection.

*Recommendation:* Most candidates innocently but mistakenly assume that they *must* use the ABOG program. As discussed previously, this is *not* true! The ABOG *Bulletin* specifies that you must simply exactly duplicate the *format* of the case list forms.

The ABOG program improves with each edition, but it is still fraught with frustrating software glitches. Worse yet, you have little control over the order of patients, categories, and procedures. These are key strategic elements.

I recommend that you construct *your own* program. Appendix D contains some tips. Not only are you in complete control of the best way to implement your strategy, but you can also optimize presentation and organization.

However, you don't have the best feel for what you want from your case list software until you get the basics down. Thus, I recommend you *start* with the ABOG software; it's usually free with a subsidy from a pharmaceutical company. You can order it from the ABOG website at **www.ABOG.org**. Don't worry which edition you purchase, as you will convert later. Start entering cases no latter than September.

After a few months you will quickly understand the limitations of that program. That's good, because now you know what you *don't want*. Now is the time, no later than January, to design your custom case list. Believe it or not, this can be accomplished in a few hours. Technical support is available from the consultants listed in Appendix D.

Remember, your examiners review your case list *before* they examine you. Your case list is your patient management DNA. The examiner's *first impression* of you is based on your case list. The money is clearly on the case list! Take the time to do it right.

### 3. I would have had my case list reviewed *before* I submitted it August 1.

*Recommendation:* After August 1, your case list is set in stone. Only later, when you begin preparing for its defense, do you sorrowfully appreciate how much easier it would have been if you had only reworded that problematic case.

I recommend tapping into your colleagues' collective wisdom. I would use local, regional, and academic clinicians (both generalists and sub-specialists). Their job is to give their recommendations on how to word each case. It is up to you to come up with the final wording for each case in order to meet your strategic objective. Chances are neither you nor your consultants have much experience in constructing case lists. It is well worth your money to have a seasoned professional review your last draft to aid in adding the finishing touches to the masterpiece.

Be forewarned. You must be organized and disciplined to pull this off. Send whatever you have of your case list to your colleagues in early May with a deadline of returning their edits back to you by mid-May. You should then send your case list to a professional consultant by early June. However, this schedule will give you time for only one major rewrite before you need to send it in to meet the August 1 deadline.

### 4. I would have started studying earlier.

*Recommendation:* These are the famous last words of all students. Remember, it has been a while since you had to buckle down and *really* study. The last time was when you were preparing for the written boards. Not only are you out of shape, but probably you have never prepared for an oral exam. It is *not* the same as a written exam.

Chapter 4, Getting Started, contains tips on how to budget your time, and Chapter 8, Studying for the Exam, suggests strategies for studying. Your priority before August 1 is that darn case list. However, if you have a November test, you really need to come out breathing fire by mid-August. If your test is later, you have a little wiggle room, but don't get lax and let precious study time dwindle.

The bottom line is, "To thine own self be true." Don't kid yourself—make an honest appraisal of what is practical, especially given your time constraints. To quote Nike, "Just do it!"

### 5. I would not have studied the pathology slides.

*Recommendation:* Interpretation of gross and microscopic pathology is no longer a distinct exam component. If a Kodachrome is shown, it most likely will be labeled with the diagnosis. If it is not, you do not lose points for not knowing the diagnosis. What is important is your ability to apply your clinical acumen in *managing* the patient with the disease in question. I wouldn't study *any* microscopic slides. If you feel compelled, review mucinous and serous cystadenocarcinoma of the ovary and endometrial hyperplasia and carcinoma. If you are ridiculously compulsive and want to eat up precious time, study the 27 slides listed in Table 3 of Chapter 8.

### 6. I would have had my case list reviewed *after* I submitted it August 1.

*Recommendation:* Now that your case list is set in stone, you must defend it. You and the consultants discussed in #3 must view your case list from the examiner's eyes and predict what kind of questions he will ask. The more sets of eyes that review your list, the more you will see a clear pattern emerging, allowing you to narrow down your list of top ten cases. Predicting your test topics will enable you to prioritize your studying, as well as focus your mock oral exams.

### 7. I should have taken a *board* review course.

*Recommendation:* Time is precious and tight. It seems like it was easier to find the time when you were a resident. Now everybody wants your time—family, practice, church, etc. Take the time to research your review courses. I recommend you find a *board* review course, which is targeted specifically to preparing you for your board exam, and not just a general review. Take into consideration how long the course is and how long you will be away from the office. Chapter 4 and Appendix H can help guide you.

Bottom line is you must step away. Few can review the volume and intensity of subjects on their own. Your studying will be made much more efficient by going to a review course. However, make sure they streamline and focus your studying to high-yield exam topics.

### 8. I should have attended a tutorial workshop.

*Recommendation:* Strategy and tactics are involved throughout the entire process. Why reinvent the wheel when you can tap into others' collective wisdom?

I recommend you take a one-day workshop on how to construct your case list. This will not only give you specific ideas to incorporate, but also get a number of pairs of eyes on your cases. By giving up only one day, you will advance toward getting to a polished product in an exponential fashion. I recommend attending only after you have some experience under your belt in working with your case list. Attend one in the late winter or spring so that you have time to incorporate the strategy.

Along that same theme, if you've never taken an oral board exam, then why take chances? Again, tap into those who have mentored many and have the expertise and feedback to give you timely tips and help. I recommend attending a one- or two-day workshop on oral exam strategy within one or two months of your exam.

### 9. I would have taken (more) mock oral exams.

*Recommendation:* The learning curve for taking an oral exam is no different from any other exponential learning curve for a new skill. When you first learned to tie surgical knots, you had to practice. This is no different, and it's actually a lot easier.

Most candidates can get to the top of the learning curve with just *three* mock orals. A pool of examiners is right at your fingertips. Just pick up the phone and call your referring MFM, oncologist, or REI. Even easier, call one of your local generalist colleagues. Have her review your case list to identify test topics. After you have studied your case list, have her give you a mock oral.

You need to get your first mock oral under your belt no later than one month before your exam. Obviously, you need to get the remaining two within the one to two weeks before the test. You definitely need to take at least one with someone who does not know you in order to remove any "home-court" bias. I recommend a faculty member at one of the review courses or the colleague of one of your referral consultants.

### 6. I would have started collecting my chief year cases sooner.

*Recommendation:* Life is unpredictable. How many knew you would end up exactly where you are today? I know it sounds crazy, but you might get an insane notion and decide to do a subspecialty fellowship. Thus, I recommend the following for **all** residents: **Hold onto your chief residency case log!** Once you know that you really will be going on to a fellowship, then begin collecting cases from your chief year in your non-fellowship discipline. Unless you stay in the same town as your residency, it is a nightmare to go back and collect cases. I recommend you begin collecting cases just as I recommended for Lessons Learned #1 on page 203. Do not put off until tomorrow what you can do today!

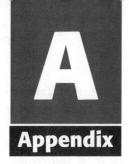

# ABOG Acceptable Case List Abbreviations

| A&P repair | Anterior and posterior colporrhaphy |
| Ab | Abortion |
| AIDS | Acquired immune deficiency syndrome |
| BS&O | Bilateral salpingo-oophorectomy |
| CD | Cesarean delivery |
| cm | Centimeter |
| D&C | Dilatation and curettage |
| D&E | Dilatation and evacuation |
| DHEA | Dehydroepiandrosterone |
| E | Estrogen |
| FSH | Follicle-stimulating hormone |
| gms | Grams |
| HIV | Human immunodeficiency virus |
| HRT | Hormone replacement therapy |
| IUD | Intrauterine device |
| kg | Kilogram |
| Pap | Papanicolaou smear |
| PROM | Premature rupture of membranes |
| PTL | Preterm labor |
| SAB | Spontaneous abortion |
| SVD | Spontaneous vaginal delivery |
| T | Testosterone |
| TAH | Total abdominal hysterectomy |
| TSH | Thyroid-stimulating hormone |
| TVH | Total vaginal hysterectomy |
| VBAC | Vaginal birth after cesarean |
| VIP | Voluntary interruption of pregnancy |

**Author's editorial comment:** Don't feel like you have to limit yourself to only these abbreviations. Your case list will not be rejected for throwing in a few that are not on this list. Just use conventional abbreviations. The columns are narrow and your case list gets cluttered with tedious long words that we conventionally abbreviate. For example, I would use DMPA rather than spelling out depot medroxyprogesterone acetate. Avoid regional colloquialism such as IOL, Induction of Labor. An easy check to make sure your abbreviation is conventional is to take your case list to the review course and get a couple of opinions from some people who are not geographically close. If everyone instantly recognizes and uses the same abbreviations, then you're set.

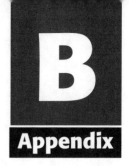

# Acronyms and Abbreviations

| | |
|---|---|
| ABC | America's OB/GYN Board Review Course |
| A&P | Anterior and posterior colporrhaphy |
| ABOG | American Board of Obstetrics and Gynecology, Inc. |
| ACOG | American College of Obstetricians and Gynecologists |
| BHCG | Beta human chorionic gonadotropin |
| BSO | Bilateral salpingo-oophorectomy |
| CD | Cesarean delivery |
| CIN | Cervical intraepithelial neoplasia |
| CMS | Center for Medicare and Medicaid Services |
| c/o | Complains of |
| CREOG | Council on Resident Education in Obstetrics and Gynecology |
| CS | Cesarean section |
| CT | Computerized tomography |
| D&C | Dilatation and curettage |
| DIC | Disseminated intravascular coagulation |
| DMPA | Depot medroxyprogesterone acetate |
| EGA | Estimated gestational age |
| EKG | Electrocardiogram |
| FACOG | Fellow of the American College of Obstetricians and Gynecologists |
| G | Gravida |
| GDM | Gestational Diabetes Mellitus |
| GnRH | Gonadotropin Releasing Hormone Agonists |
| GNS | General Surgeon |
| GYN | Gynecology |
| HCG | Human chorionic gonadotropin |
| HIPAA | Health Insurance Portability and Accounting Act of 1996 |
| HMOs | Health maintenance organizations |
| HPV | Human papilloma virus |
| HRT | Hormone replacement therapy |
| HSV | Herpes simplex virus |
| HTN | Hypertension |

| | |
|---|---|
| IC | Interstitial cystitis |
| IUPC | Intrauterine pressure catheter |
| JC | Joint Commission |
| LAVH | Laparoscopic assisted vaginal hysterectomy |
| LMP | Last menstrual period |
| LSH | Laparoscopic supracervical hysterectomy |
| MFM | Maternal fetal medicine specialist |
| MOC | Maintenance of Certification |
| MRI | Magnetic resonance imaging |
| NSAIDs | Nonsteroidal anti-inflammatory drugs |
| OAB | Overactive bladder |
| OB | Obstetrics |
| OCPs | Oral contraceptive pills |
| P | Parity |
| PACU | Post-anesthesia care unit |
| PAR | Post-anesthesia recovery room |
| PID | Pelvic inflammatory disease |
| PMP | Postmenopausal |
| PPTL | Postpartum tubal ligation |
| PPROM | Preterm prolonged rupture of membranes |
| PROM | Prolonged rupture of membranes |
| POD | Postoperative day |
| REI | Reproductive endocrinology infertility |
| RR | Recovery room |
| SCIP | Surgical Care Improvement Project |
| SIL | Squamous intraepithelial lesion |
| SOB | Shortness of breath |
| S/P | Status post |
| SPVT | Septic pelvic vein thrombosis |
| SROM | Spontaneous rupture of membranes |
| STD | Sexually transmitted disease |
| SUI | Stress urinary incontinence |
| TAH | Total abdominal hysterectomy |
| TLH | Total laparoscopic hysterectomy |
| TVH | Transvaginal or total vaginal hysterectomy |
| UI | Urinary incontinence |
| U/S | Ultrasound |
| UTI | Urinary tract infection |
| VBAC | Vaginal birth after cesarean section |
| VH | Vaginal hysterectomy |
| VIN | Vulvar intraepithelial neoplasia |
| V/Q | Ventilation-perfusion scan |

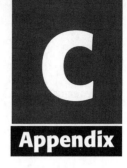

**Appendix**

# Addresses

American Board of Obstetrics and Gynecology, Inc.
   2915 Vine Street, Suite 300
   Dallas, TX 75204-1069
   Phone: (214) 871-1619
   Fax: (214) 871-1943
   e-mail: info@abog.org
   http://www.abog.org

American College of Obstetricians and Gynecologists
   409 12th Street, S.W.
   P.O. Box 96920
   Washington, DC 20090-6920
   Phone: (202) 638-5577
   1-800-673-8444
   Fax: (202) 484-5107
   e-mail: use initial of first name followed by up to seven
   characters of the last name followed by @acog.com
   http://www.acog.org

For publications: ACOG Distribution Center, 1-800-762-2264 or
http://www.acog.org

America's OB/GYN Board Review Course
  PO Box 1126
  Hendersonville, NC 28793
  Phone: 1-877-ABC-OBGYN (1-877-222-6249)
  FAX: (828) 698-5510
  e-mail: info@americasboardreview.com
  http://www.americasboardreview.com

Author of This Book
  A. Krishna Das, MD, FACOG
  622 Sabine Drive
  Hendersonville, NC 28739
  Phone: (828) 698-9220
  Cellular phone: (828) 606-6956
  Fax: (828) 687-1814
  e-mail: krisdas@earthlink.net  or  krisdas@mchsi.com

Case List Consultant
  Janine Keever, MD, FACOG
  64 Eastgate Drive
  Sylva, NC 27834
  Phone: 1-877-ABC-OBGYN (1-877-222-6249)
  Office : (828) 631-1960
  e-mail: DrKeever@yahoo.com

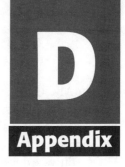

# Appendix D

# Custom Case List

The most influential factor for passing your test is your case list. Henceforth, it is imperative that you strategically construct it to put your best foot forward. Remember, your examiner sees your case list before he even shakes your hand; therefore, his first impression of you is based entirely on your case list.

Your priority then is to construct the best case list possible. It is absolutely imperative that you select the case list software that will best help you meet your goals. You have two options. You can either purchase pre-existing case list software or create your own. Let's review the pros and cons of each.

## ABOG Software

ABOG has a CD that you may obtain by simply calling, writing, or going online to ABOG (per Appendix C). Candidates *erroneously* assume that it is mandatory that they use the ABOG software. This is simply not true. You may use **any** format, as long as it *exactly* duplicates the ABOG case list forms.

The ABOG software is the least preferable option, in my opinion. ACOG was the first to author the software in the early 1990s and relinquished this to ABOG in the early 2000s. As with any project, each revision improves; however, it continues to have many limitations.

The ABOG program is not very user friendly. You have little control of the order of cases and editing within each case. The ABOG software will not let you easily make logical word breaks in columns or pages, nor can you align your flow of thought from one column to the next. Finally, the ABOG software doesn't track statistics accurately for your summary sheets.

The overall impression is inferior compared to the other options. An ABOG-generated case list does not present as well and is not optimal in strategic construction. Consistently, a chief regret of past candidates is using the ABOG software. Unfortunately, since you have not reviewed many case lists, if any, you have to trust me on this. All I can say is that after having reviewed hundreds of case lists over more than nearly two decades, a well-constructed case list is truly **outstanding** compared to the majority that settle for mediocrity.

Take my word, as well as your colleagues': **Don't** start with the ABOG software. By the time you realize your errors, it's harder, though not impossible, to turn back and start over again.

So if not the ABOG program, then what? You have two remaining options: purchase a different commercial software or create your own. The obvious disadvantage of the latter is that it is more time consuming and requires proficiency in formatting.

## Commercial Software

There are a number of commercial software products available. Most are better than the ABOG software, so you end up with a better product. However, like any software designed by someone else, you are again subject to their rules, biases, and formatting. Thus, your case list will look like all the others that have used the same software, so ironically you're right back to the problem of blending in with the rest of the crowd.

Additionally, commercial products can be costly compared to the ABOG program, which is usually free, as it is usually subsidized by an educational grant. Furthermore, you must be careful that the software is up-to-date and reflects the latest ABOG changes. Remember, your case list format must *exactly* reproduce that required by ABOG. If you are a Mac user, I am not aware of any software written for the Mac at this time. You may, however, draft a customized case list, as discussed below.

## Customized Case List

Your final option is to create your own case list program. This is clearly the most time consuming, but also assures your case list will conform entirely to *your* standard. **No one** will have a case list that looks like yours. You **will** stand out.

The best case list I have **ever** seen was that from a candidate nearing retirement! I had two questions for him: 1) "Why on earth are you taking the test now?" and 2) "How did/could you construct such a beautiful case list?"

His response to my first question was that was something he wanted to do for himself before he died. Many years ago, there was not the emphasis nor the mandate for board certification as there is now. He never needed board certification to practice, but he prided himself on always keeping up to date. This was his last validation of a successful career… and something he wanted to quietly achieve for himself.

His response to my second question was quite simple. His *high school* son created the case list! His son was entering the data in the then ACOG software. It had so many glitches that he, *on his own*, created the custom software!

For most of you, you're of the same generation as his son (born since the 1980s), so you can easily do the same. I was lecturing at a review course on this topic and showed the audience an example of the above case list. Barbara Dill, MD, approached me the **next** day with a draft of her attempt. It was good, but I felt it could be better. To make a long story short, it took her only three consecutive evenings to program a stellar case list. I have had this same story repeated time after time. Literally, designing the template takes just a few hours. Here's how.

## Paradigm Shift

Recall in Chapter 5, The Case List, and Chapter 9, Image Enhancement, that we discussed the necessity to step out of your shoes and into the examiner's. You need to undergo a paradigm shift and look at your case list as if you were the examiner.

Pick up yours or anybody's case list. What cases would you ask about? *Why* would you ask about those cases? Chances are because it was an interesting or unusual topic or perhaps because of the complication that ensued.

Whatever the reason, you can use this to your advantage by simply making that word(s) stand out and catch your eye. You can **bold**, CAPITALIZE, <u>underline</u>, or *italicize* that key word. How about even highlighting or shading the whole column? Physically changing the keyword or phrase will pull the eye involuntarily to that word. **Gotcha**! Now the examiner may acknowledge that yes, indeed, this is something that he would like to ask about. And you are ready for him, because you set the bait.

Remember, many of your examiners are over forty and wear bifocals. ABOG mandates that the size of the print be at least 12-point. How about carrying that a step further? Your software should give you the freedom to organize to your choosing. You can insert horizontal tracking lines to follow the flow within and between columns. Consider leaving a space between patients. Place vertical tracking lines to demarcate columns. A most elegant organizational tool is bullets. Will your software allow you to insert them?

Finally, make sure your software allows you ease in editing. You shouldn't have to struggle and redo the whole page just to add or delete words. Also, you must be able to control where your word breaks when carrying over within a column. An absolute no-no is carrying over a case when the page breaks.

If I've persuaded you at least philosophically to consider customizing your case list, then the next step is logistics. Believe it or not, this is the easy and rewarding part.

## Software

Obviously, there are a number of software products on the market. You should choose the one that you are the most comfortable with, as well as that which is the most capable of producing the desired product. The most common are Microsoft Word or Microsoft Excel.

My preference for a customized case list is Microsoft Word. Although it is primarily utilized for entering and editing straight text, it has significant formatting muscle that can help make your case list outstanding. You will read below what pertinent heading information and categories must be included in each section of the case list. Since each section of the case list is a bit different, you will need three different formatted documents, one for each of the Obstetrics, Gynecology and Office Practices cases. Don't fret! Once you get one of them figured out, the other case list sections are easily applied.

The first part of your Word document is to create a header with the mandatory information at the top of each page. This includes the page number, your name, case list number and whether these are post-residency, fellowship or senior residency cases. You can also include in the header the column titles for that specific section. For example, on your Office Practice case list, you would include everything from patient number through the number of patient visits.

Your two biggest challenges will be to choose an acceptable font that you can easily read, yet also make your margins small enough to fit everything. Now you need to decide on left or center alignments, as well as top and bottom alignments for each column heading. That's it! Since this is now in your Word header, it will appear on every page of your case list automatically.

The second part of your Word document will be the actual body of the document. Now create a table that lines up exactly with the column headings that you just created in your header. If your header has 15 columns, then so will your main content in the body of the document. Once that is done, you are ready to start entering data.

I would recommend trying out just three or four cases to see how it will look before you dive into your data entry. Basically, each case is a new row in your table. By entering a few cases, you will then be able to experiment with the other types of formatting options. Should you use bullets? What do you want them to look like? Where do you want to use them? Which fonts look better? How can you best clarify your patient management?

Furthermore, you can insert a new row for each of your categories. A snazzy look is to then merge the cells in that row so it can fit all the way across. To make a new area stand out even more, you can use light colored shading in that new row, or perhaps bold your chosen font for the category headings. You will have to see what is pleasing to your eye, although I would recommend staying on the conservative side when it comes to shading.

You can apply the same methods to Excel. The advantage is that the Excel worksheet is already a table. However, I feel the formatting options for text is not as viable.

Regardless, whichever program you decide to create your case list, have fun with it and let the creative juices flow! Just remember to stay within the minimal guidelines laid out by ABOG.

## Setting Up Your Own Database

Creating your database or template is the biggest challenge. Once it is set, making the case list is simply a matter of data entry. Your database must comply exactly with the ABOG specifications. Check the ABOG website for the most up-to-date forms. Your initial packet from ABOG includes these specifications as well as sample pages for the three sections (Examples 1, 2, and 3), the summary sheet (Examples 4, 5 and 6), and the affidavit sheet (see below).

Each page of the case list has a heading (List of Obstetric Patients, List of Gynecologic Patients, or List of Office Practice Patients), page number, your name, case list number and whether they are post-residency, fellowship or senior residency cases. Each section (Obstetrics, Gynecology, or Office) has specific columns to list each case. Each respective section (OB, GYN, or Office) should begin with page number 1 and be numbered consecutively thereafter. Furthermore, each patient should be numbered consecutively so that every patient has a unique number as well. Refer to Chapter 5 for a list of categories for each section. If you do not have a patient in one of the categories, still list the category heading, but specify "None" on the form.

---

**AFFIDAVIT SHEET FOR EACH SITE**

Candidate's Name: _____

Hospital: _____

Hospital Address: _____

           Street          City, State         Zip Code

ATTEST:  The patients listed on pages _____ through _____ include ALL
hospitalized patients discharged or transferred from the care of
DOCTOR _____
at this hospital (site) from _____
               to_____
                      (Date)

Signature and Title of Hospital (site) Official
(e.g., Medical Record Administrator or Other): _____
                     (Signature)

                     (Title)

Signature of the Candidate: _____

**The American Board of Obstetrics and Gynecology reserves the right to audit the accuracy of this list.**

**Obstetrical Case List Forms**

☐ Post Residency Cases   ☐ Senior Residency Cases   ☐ Fellowship Cases

LIST OF OBSTETRICAL PATIENTS*

| # | HOSP # | PAT # | AGE # | GRAV # | PARA | Gest Age | COMPLICATIONS | | Operative Procedures And/or Treatment | Days In Hosp. (Not Dates) | NEWBORN | | | |
|---|---|---|---|---|---|---|---|---|---|---|---|---|---|---|
| | | | | | | | Antepartum | Delivery or Postpartum | | | Perinatal Death | Wgt | APGAR 1 & 5 Minutes | Days In Hosp. (Not Dates) |

I.   Number of Uncomplicated Spontaneous Deliveries _____
II.  Obstetrical Categories (1-31) _____
III. Total number of <u>ultrasound</u> and <u>Color Doppler examinations</u> performed by you upon hospitalized obstetrical patients _____
IV.  Total number of:
    A.  APGAR scores 5 or less _____
    B.  Infants < 2500 gms _____
    C.  Perinatal Deaths _____

\* Patients' names, initials, and hospital names must not be used.  Also, patients who are over 89 years of age must not have their age listed.

\# refers to a sequential ordering which is assigned by the computer for ALL patients from all hospitals, i.e., 1-xxx.

**Hospital #** refers to the sequential ordering of hospitals being reported from, i.e., reported;

    Hospital A = First hospital from which patients are being reported;
    Hospital B = Second hospital from which patients are being reported;
    Hospital C = Third hospital from which patients are being reported.

Patient # refers to a sequential ordering of patients reported from a given hospital, i.e., Hospital A, patients 1-x; Hospital B, patients 1-xx.

**Example 1**

**Gynecological Case List Forms**

□ Post Residency Cases    □ Senior Residency Cases    □ Fellowship Cases

| LIST OF GYNECOLOGICAL PATIENTS* | | | | | | | | | |
|---|---|---|---|---|---|---|---|---|---|
| HOSP # | PAT # | AGE | GRAV | PARA | DIAGNOSIS PREOPERATIVE OR ADMISSION | TREATMENT | SURGICAL PATHOLOGY DIAGNOSIS (Uterine Wt. in gms.) | COMPLICATIONS (Include blood transfusions) | Days In Hosp. (Not Dates) |

i.   Gynecological Categories (1-29)

II.  Total number of <u>ultrasound</u> and <u>Color Doppler Examinations</u> performed by you upon hospitalized gynecological patients _____

\* Patients' names, initials, and hospital names must not be used. Also, patients who are over 89 years of age must not have their age listed.

\# refers to a sequential ordering which is assigned by the computer for ALL patients from all hospitals, i.e., 1-xxx.

**Hospital #** refers to the sequential ordering of hospitals being reported from, i.e., Hospital A = First hospital from which patients are being reported; Hospital B = Second hospital from which patients are being reported; Hospital C = Third hospital from which patients are being reported.

**Patient #** refers to a sequential ordering of patients reported from a given hospital, i.e., Hospital A, patients 1-x; Hospital B, patients 1-xx.

**Example 2**

**Office Practice Case List Forms**

LIST OF OFFICE PRACTICE PATIENTS*

| # | A G E | G R A V | P A R A | PROBLEM | DIAGNOSTIC PROCEDURES | TREATMENT | RESULTS | No. of Visits |
|---|---|---|---|---|---|---|---|---|
| | | | | | | | | |

I. Office Practice Categories (1-40)
II. Total Number of <u>Ultrasound and Color Doppler Examinations</u> in:
   A, Obstetrical patients _____
   B. Gynecological patients _____
   C. Other areas such as abdominal, thoracic, pediatric, etc. _____

* Patient's names, initials and hospital names must not be used. Also, patients who are over 89 years of age must not have their age listed.

# refers to a sequential ordering which is assigned by the computer for ALL patients from all hospitals, i.e., 1-xxx.

The American Board of Obstetrics and Gynecology offers a case list collection and reporting software program for the oral examination (available on-line or email caselists@abog.org or phone 214 871-1619)

**Example 3**

Candidate's Name _____     Case List ID # _____     Date Range of Case List _____

## SUMMARY SHEET/ALL HOSPITALS AND AMBULATORY SURGICAL SITES COMBINED

| A. GYNECOLOGIC CATEGORIES | Total Cases | Total Applied |
|---|---|---|
| Abdominal Hysterectomy | | |
| Laparotomy (Other than Tubal Sterilization) | | |
| Vaginal Hysterectomy (Including Laparoscopically Assisted) | | |
| Diagnostic Laparoscopy | | |
| Operative Laparoscopy (Other than Tubal Sterilization) | | |
| Operative Hysteroscopy | | |
| Uterine Myomas | | |
| Defects in Pelvic Floor | | |
| Endometriosis | | |
| Tubal Sterilization | | |
| Invasive Carcinoma | | |
| Carcinoma in situ | | |
| Infertility Evaluation | | |
| Infertility Treatment | | |
| Urinary Incontinence | | |
| Urinary Incontinence (Surgical Treatment) | | |
| Ectopic Pregnancy | | |
| Abdominal Hysterectomy | | |
| Pelvic Pain | | |
| Congenital Abnormalities of the Reproductive Tract | | |
| Pelvic Inflammatory Disease | | |
| Adnexal Problems excluding Ectopic Pregnancy and Pelvic Inflammatory Disease | | |
| Abnormal Uterine Bleeding | | |
| Vulvar Masses | | |
| Vulvar Ulcers | | |
| Adenomyosis | | |

| A. GYNECOLOGIC CATEGORIES | Total Cases | Total Applied |
|---|---|---|
| Postoperative Wound Complications | | |
| Postoperative Thrombophlebitis and/or Embolism | | |
| Postoperative Fever for Greater than 48 hours | | |
| Rectovaginal or Urinary Tract Fistula | | |
| Culposcopy | | |
| TOTAL CASES | | |

B. NUMBER OF HOSPITAL STAYS > 7 DAYS

C. GYNECOLOGIC ULTRASOUNDS & DOPPLER EXAMINATIONS

**Example 4**

Candidate's Name

Case List ID #

Date Range of Case List

## SUMMARY SHEET/ALL HOSPITALS AND AMBULATORY SURGICAL SITES COMBINED

| A. OBSTETRIC CATEGORIES | Total Cases | Total Applied |
|---|---|---|
| Breech and Other Fetal Malpresentations | | |
| Intrapartum Infection (Amnionitis) | | |
| Puerperal Infection | | |
| Third Trimester Bleeding | | |
| Multifetal Pregnancy | | |
| Cesarean Pregnancy | | |
| Premature Rupture of Fetal Membranes at Term | | |
| Preterm Premature Rupture of Membranes | | |
| Preterm Delivery | | |
| Hypertensive Disorders of Pregnancy (Chronic hypertension, preeclampsia, eclampsia) | | |
| Second Trimester Spontaneous Abortion | | |
| Cardiovascular and/or Pulmonary Diseases Complicating Pregnancy | | |
| Renal Diseases and/or Neurological Diseases Complicating Pregnancy | | |
| Hematological Disease and/or Endocrine Diseases Complicating Pregnancy | | |
| Infections Complicating Pregnancy | | |
| Postterm Pregnancy | | |
| Abnormal Fetal Growth | | |
| Vaginal Birth After Cesarean Delivery | | |
| Any Maternal Complication which Delayed Maternal Hospital Discharge by 48 or More Hours | | |
| Any Neonatal Complication which Delayed Neonatal Hospital Discharge by 48 or More Hours | | |
| Pregnancies Complicated by Fetal Anomalies | | |

| A. OBSTETRIC CATEGORIES | Total Cases | Total Applied |
|---|---|---|
| Pregnancies Complicated by Human Immunodeficiency Virus Infection (HIV) | | |
| Primary Cesarean Delivery | | |
| Repeat Cesarean Delivery | | |
| Inductions and/or Augmentations of Labor | | |
| Puerpal Hemorrhage | | |
| Readmission for Maternal Complication Up to 6 Weeks Postpartum | | |
| **TOTAL CASES** | | |
| B. TOTAL UNCOMPLICATED SPONTANEOUS DELIVERIES | | |
| C. OBSTETRIC ULTRASOUNDS & DOPPLER EXAMINATIONS | | |
| D. NUMBER OF OTHER OBSTETRICAL CONSIDERATIONS | | |
|    1. Apgar Scores 5 or less | | |
|    2. Infants < 2500 gms | | |
|    3. Perinatal deaths | | |

**Example 5**

225

Candidate's Name | Case List ID # | Date Range of Case List

## SUMMARY SHEET/ALL HOSPITALS AND AMBULATORY SURGICAL SITES COMBINED

| A. OFFICE PRACTICE CATEGORIES | Total Cases | Total Applied | A. OFFICE PRACTICE CATEGORIES | Total Cases | Total Applied |
|---|---|---|---|---|---|
| Preventive Care and Health Maintenance | | | Spousal Abuse | | |
| Counseling for Smoking Cessation and Treatment of Obesity | | | Dysmenorrhea | | |
| Counseling for Sexual Dysfunction | | | Premenstrual Syndrome | | |
| Contraception | | | Benign Pelvic Masses | | |
| Psychosomatic Problems | | | Vaginal Ultrasonography | | |
| Genetic Counseling | | | Back Pain | | |
| Primary or Secondary Amenorrhea | | | Respiratory Tract Diseases | | |
| Hirsutism | | | Gastrointestinal Diseases | | |
| Infertility | | | Cardiovascular Diseases | | |
| Hyperprolactinemia | | | Endocrine Diseases (Diabetes Mellitus, Thyroid or Adrenal Disease) | | |
| Endometriosis | | | Hypertension | | |
| Menopausal Care | | | Diagnosis and Management of Hypercholesterolemia and Dyslipidemias | | |
| Office Surgery | | | Recognition and Counseling for Substance Abuse (Alcohol, Narcotics, etc.) | | |
| Abnormal Uterine Bleeding | | | Depression | | |
| Abnormal Cervical Cytology | | | Geriatrics | | |
| Pelvic Pain | | | | | |
| Vaginal Discharge | | | | | |
| Vulvar Disease | | | | | |
| Breast Diseases | | | | | |
| Urinary Incontinence and Pelvic Floor Defects | | | | | |
| Urinary Tract Infections | | | | | |
| Sexually Transmitted Diseases | | | | | |
| Preconceptional Counseling | | | | | |
| Immunizations | | | | | |
| Pediatric Gynecology | | | | | |
| Sexual Assault | | | | | |

**Example 6**

## Setting Up Your Obstetric Database

The obstetric list is subcategorized into Number of Uncomplicated Spontaneous Deliveries, Obstetrical Categories, Total Number of Ultrasound and Color Doppler Examinations Performed by You Upon Hospitalized Obstetrical Patients, and Total number of Apgar scores of 5 or less, Infants < 2500 grams, and Perinatal Deaths. You can make the categories stand out by shadowing the title (Example 7). The column headings are as follows:

| | |
|---|---|
| Patient's case list number | Operative procedures and/or treatment |
| Patient's hospital number | Patient's number of days in the hospital |
| Age | Newborn perinatal death |
| Gravida | Newborn weight |
| Parity | Apgars at 1 and 5 minutes |
| Gestational age | Newborn days in hospital |
| Complications of antepartum | |
| Complications of delivery or postpartum | |

The most challenging part of designing your obstetric list is to fit all the columns on one page. As more information is entered, the print becomes smaller and more difficult to read. Try the following tricks to make this section look its best:

1. Make the left and right margins as wide as possible and narrow the non-complication columns.

2. Use a large, easy-on-the-eye font. (ABOG mandates a minimum of 12 points.) Experiment with different ones until you find one you like.

3. List the required information vertically rather than horizontally within a column to save space and, more importantly, to align flow of thought between columns. Using formatting bullets will help you with vertical listing. Draw a horizontal line between cases. Limit each page to six or so cases; a longer list results in eye strain and overwhelms the reader with too much data (compare Example 8 with Example 9).

## LIST OF OBSTETRIC PATIENTS

Page 1

July 1, _____ —June 30, _____

Candidate's name _____

| # | Initials & Hosp. No. | Age | Gravida | Para | Gest. Age | Complications — Antepartum | Complications — Delivery or Postpartum | Opertive Procedures and/or Treatment | Days in Hosp. | Newborn Complications | Wgt. (gm) | Apgar 1 & 5 Minutes | Days in Hosp. |
|---|---|---|---|---|---|---|---|---|---|---|---|---|---|
| A. Antepartum Admissions | | | | | | | | | | | | | |
| | | | | | | | | | | | | | |
| B. Obstetric Deliveries | | | | | | | | | | | | | |
| | | | | | | | | | | | | | |
| C. Other Obstetric Considerations | | | | | | | | | | | | | |
| | | | | | | | | | | | | | |
| D. Postpartum Readmissions | | | | | | | | | | | | | |
| | | | | | | | | | | | | | |
| E. Patients Transfused | | | | | | | | | | | | | |
| | | | | | | | | | | | | | |
| Total Normal, Uncomplicated Obstetric Patients | | | | | | | | | | | | | |
| Total Number of Ultrasound and Doppler Examinations on Hospitalized Obstetric Patients | | | | | | | | | | | | | |

**Example 7**

## LIST OF OBSTETRIC PATIENTS

Barbara Angelika Dill, M.D.

| # Initials & Hosp. No. | Age | Gravida | Para | Gest. Age | Complications — Antepartum | Complications — Delivery or Postpartum | Operative Procedures and/or Treatment | Days Hosp. | Newborn Complications | Wgt. | Apgar 1 & 5 Minutes | Days Hosp. |
|---|---|---|---|---|---|---|---|---|---|---|---|---|
| MR 646681 | 24 | 2 | 1011 | 40 | Anorexia nervosa | | PG cervical ripening / Pitocin induction / SVD | 2 | | 3575 gm | 9 & 10 | 2 |
| DB 652108 | 20 | 3 | 2012 | 41 | Post-dates | | Pitocin induction / SVD | 2 | | 3305 gm | 8 & 9 | 2 |
| AP 649784 | 37 | 3 | 1021 | 36 | Advanced maternal age / PROM | | Amniocentesis @ 15 wk / Pitocin induction / SVD | 2 | | 2635 gm | 9 & 10 | 2 |
| MS 643860 | 28 | 2 | 1011 | 40 | Abnor. triple screen (high AFP) / First-trimester bleeding / Meconium | | Amniocentesis @ 19 wk / Low forceps delivery | 2 | | 2810 gm | 9 & 9 | 2 |
| MM 652021 | 31 | 4 | 3013 | 40 | Previous CD, requesting VBAC | | PG cervical ripening / Pitocin induction / VBAC / Postpartum tubal ligation | 3 | | 2970 gm | 9 & 10 | 2 |
| AC 498963 | 24 | 5 | 2122 | 39 | Previous PROM × 2 / PROM | | Pitocin induction / SVD / Postpartum tubal ligation | 2 | | 3625 gm | 9 & 9 | 2 |
| SI 650218 | 20 | 1 | 1 | 39 | PROM × 24 hr | | Pitocin induction | 2 | Mild hypospadias | 2745 gm | 9 & 10 | 2 |
| MF 652336 | 20 | 1 | 1 | 38 | PROM × 36 hr / Suspected chorioamnionitis / Late decelerations | | Antibiotic prophylaxis / Pitocin augmentation / Cesarean section | 4 | | 3941 gm | 8 & 9 | 4 |
| LR 471681 | 30 | 4 | 3013 | 39 | | | SVD / Postpartum tubal ligation | 2 | | 3235 gm | 9 & 10 | 2 |
| EM 650386 | 24 | 2 | 1011 | 39 | | | Pitocin induction / Outlet forceps delivery | 2 | | 3605 gm | 9 & 9 | 2 |
| NW 597958 | 28 | 1 | 1 | 36 | | | Antibiotic prophylaxis / Vacuum delivery | 2 | | 3190 gm | 9 & 10 | 2 |
| KP 636620 | 20 | 3 | 1021 | 39 | Bicornuate uterus on sono / First-trimester bleeding / Breech in labor | | CD | 4 | | 2765 gm | 9 & 10 | 4 |
| MG 652694 | 30 | 2 | 2 | 38 | | Abnor. placenta (wt. 455 gm) / Velamentous cord insertion / 30% placental infarction / Cord avuls. & retained placenta | SVD / Manual delivery of placenta / Postpartum curettage / Postpartum tubal ligation | 2 | | 2260 gm | 9 & 10 | 2 |

**Example 8**

## LIST OF OBSTETRIC PATIENTS

Barbara Angelika Dill, M.D.

Page 4
July 1, 1996–June 30, 1997
Hospital Site: Englewood Hospital

| # | Initials & Hosp. No. | Age | Gravida | Para | Gest. Age | Complications Antepartum | Complications Delivery or Postpartum | Opertive Procedures and/or Treatment | Days Hosp. | Newborn Complications | Wgt. (gm) | Apgar 1 & 5 Minutes | Days Hosp. |
|---|---|---|---|---|---|---|---|---|---|---|---|---|---|
| 22 | SD 644413 | 27 | 3 | 2 | 39 | Pregnancy-induced hypertension | None | Pitocin induction<br>SVD<br>Postpartum tubal ligation | 2 | None | 3525 | 9 & 10 | 2 |
| 23 | VW 651545 | 34 | 2 | 1 | 38 | Inadequate expulsive forces due to maternal exhaustion | Postpartum depression | Pitocin augmentation<br>Low forceps delivery | 2 | Baby kept by DYFS | 3185 | 9 & 10 | 7 |
| 24 | BB 644567 | 36 | 3 | 2 | 39 | Prior CD requesting VBAC | None | PG cervical ripening<br>Pitocin induction<br>VBAC | 2 | None | 3850 | 8 & 8 | 2 |
| 25 | MR 646681 | 24 | 2 | 1 | 40 | Anorexia nervosa | None | PG cervical ripening<br>Pitocin induction<br>SVD | 2 | None | 3575 | 9 & 10 | 2 |
| 26 | DB 652108 | 20 | 3 | 1 | 41 | Post-dates | None | Pitocin induction<br>SVD | 2 | None | 3305 | 8 & 9 | 2 |
| 27 | AP 649784 | 37 | 3 | 0 | 36 | PROM<br>Maternal age > 35, norm. amniocentesis | None | Pitocin induction<br>SVD | 2 | None | 2635 | 9 & 10 | 2 |
| 28 | MS 643860 | 28 | 2 | 0 | 40 | Variable decelerations<br>Meconium<br>Abnor. triple screen, norm. amniocentesis | None | Outlet forceps delivery | 2 | None | 2810 | 9 & 9 | 2 |
| 29 | MM 652021 | 31 | 4 | 2 | 40 | Prior CD, requesting VBAC | None | PG cervical ripening<br>Pitocin induction<br>VBAC<br>Postpartum tubal ligation | 3 | None | 2970 | 9 & 10 | 2 |

**Example 9**

## Setting Up Your Gynecologic Database

The gynecologic case list is subcategorized into the categories listed on the summary sheet. The column headings are as follows:

| | |
|---|---|
| Patient's case list number | Diagnosis (preoperative or admission) |
| Patient's hospital number | Treatment |
| Patient's number | Surgical pathology diagnosis |
| Age | Complications |
| Gravida | Number of days hospitalized |
| Parity | |

Because there are fewer columns than on the obstetric case list, it is easier to fit all data on one page. However, the same recommendations to enhance readability apply. Remember to start over on the page count and the patient numbering. Do not forget to include size (cm) for ovarian cysts, weight (grams) for uterine pathology and blood transfusions for complications. Examples 10 and 11 are ideal in presentation and content.

Notice the proper use of bullets, cases per page, and abbreviations.

## LIST OF GYNECOLOGIC PATIENTS

1 July 1996–30 June 1997
Page 4

Candidate's Name:  John Q. Doe

Hospital or Site Name:  Bridgeport Hospital

List ALL gynecology patients in each hospital or clinical site in the following order:
I. Hospitalized patients: A. Major operative procedures, B. Minor operative procedures, C. Nonsurgical admissions, D. Total number of ultrasound and Doppler examinations performed by you upon hospitalized gynecologic patients.
II. Ambulatory or Short-stay surgery gynecology patients.

| # | Initials & Hosp. No. | Age | Gravida | Para | Diagnosis Preoperative or Admission (include size of ovarian cysts) | Treatment | Surgical Pathology Diagnosis (uterine wt. in gms.) | Complications (include blood transfusions) | Days in Hosp. |
|---|---|---|---|---|---|---|---|---|---|
| | TM 250906 | 33 | 0 | 0 | • Stage IV endometriosis • Failure to control pain with 3 prior laparoscopies and medical management | • TAH/BSO • Extensive lysis of adhesions | • Endometriosis • Adenomyosis • Weight—121 gm | • Vaginal cuff abscess | 4 |
| | | | | | • Postoperative vaginal cuff abscess | • Colpotomy, drainage and culture • Intravenous antibiotics | • Mixed anaerobes | • None | 2 |
| **B. Minor Operative Procedures** | | | | | | | | | |
| | CB 048942 | 50 | 2 | 2 | • Anemia, ascites, alcoholism • Consulted for presumed menometrorrhagia | • Pad count • Endometrial biopsy • Consulted for presumed menometrorrhagia | • Proliferative endometrium | • None | 12 |
| **C. Nonsurgical Admissions** | | | | | | | | | |
| | DR 127386 | 32 | 4 | 3 | • Ectopic pregnancy treated with methotrexate 4 days prior to admission • Worsening pain | • Close observation • Serial blood counts • Serial quantitative HCG | • N/A | • None | 1 |

**Example 10**

LIST OF GYNECOLOGIC PATIENTS

1 July 1996–30 June 1997
Page 4

Candidate's Name: _____

Hospital Name: _____

| # | Initials & Hosp. No. | Age | Gravida | Para | Diagnosis Preoperative or Admission (include size of ovarian cysts) | Treatment | Surgical Pathology Diagnosis (uterine wt. in gms.) | Complications (include blood transfusions) | Days in Hosp. |
|---|---|---|---|---|---|---|---|---|---|
| 1 | D.H. 601512 | 44 | 4 | 4 | • Menorrhagia • Right adnexal mass: 6 × 7 cm | • TAH—BS&O | • Uterine wt.—184 gm • Adenomyosis • Right ovary: papillary serous cyst adenoma • Left ovary: benign | None | 2 |

B. Other Laparotomies

| # | Initials & Hosp. No. | Age | Gravida | Para | Diagnosis Preoperative or Admission (include size of ovarian cysts) | Treatment | Surgical Pathology Diagnosis (uterine wt. in gms.) | Complications (include blood transfusions) | Days in Hosp. |
|---|---|---|---|---|---|---|---|---|---|
| 2 | T.G. 361206 | 29 | 3 | 1 | • Acute abdomen • Rule out ruptured ectopic pregnancy | • Laparotomy • Right salpingectomy | • Ectopic tubal gestation • Hematosalpinx • Hemoperitoneum | Anemia | 2 |
| 3 | J.F. 904281 | 27 | 4 | 1 | • Rule out ectopic pregnancy | • Diagnostic laparoscopy • Laparotomy • Right cornual pregnancy | • Right tubal pregnancy | Anemia | 2 |
| 4. | J.E. 675902 | 37 | 6 | 3 | • Missed Ab • Rule out ectopic pregnancy | • Suction D&C • Diagnostic laparoscopy • Laparotomy • Right salpingectomy | • Right tubal pregnancy | None | 2 |

**Example 11**

233

## Setting Up Your Office Practice Database

The office practice case list has 40 categories to choose from (see Chapter 5). You may list only 40 patients and no more than two patients per category. List all 40 categories but annotate "None observed" when appropriate. The ABOG program does not list the category if there are no representative patients. You are prone to then forget about these categories since "out of sight is out of mind," yet you will still be accountable for all 40 categories. Because there are fewer columns, it is very easy to include all the information on one page. Remember to reset the page number and the patient numbering. Example 12 is an excellent representation of a cleanly designed list.

The column headings are as follows:

| | |
|---|---|
| Patient's number | Problem |
| Age | Diagnostic procedures |
| Gravida | Treatment |
| Parity | Results |
| Number of patient visits | |

If you have more specific questions on how to create a custom case list, I recommend you consult Dr. Janine Keever (See Appendix C for contact information). She is the clever one who was easily and artfully able to customize her own case list.

In conclusion, you have three software options to enter your data: use ABOG's, use another commercial product, or design your own. Although all meet the ABOG criteria, the customized software will most likely result in a polished product that stands out from the rest. Given that half of the exam is based on the case list and your case list makes the first impression, seize the opportunity to use this to your complete advantage.

## LIST OF OUTPATIENTS

Barbara Angelika Dill, M.D.

July 1, 1996–June 30, 1997

| # | Initials | Age | Gravida | Para | Problem | Diagnostic Procedures | Treatment | Results | No. of Visits |
|---|----------|-----|---------|------|---------|-----------------------|-----------|---------|---------------|
| **I. Patient List** | | | | | | | | | |
| **Preoperative Care & Health Maintenance** | | | | | | | | | |
| 153 | RA | 35 | 3 | 2 | Annual exam Polycystic overy disease | Pap, baseline mammogram, lipid profile, 2h glucose test | Dietary modification | Elevated cholesterol Glucose normal | 2 |
| 154 | AG | 73 | 0 | 0 | Annual exam Breast cancer × 1 yr on tamoxifen Vaginal pruritus | Pap Endometrial biopsy: atrophic | Topical estrogen (discussed with breast surgeon and oncologist) | Resolution | 3 |
| **Obesity** | | | | | | | | | |
| None observed | | | | | | | | | |
| **Sexual Dysfunction** | | | | | | | | | |
| 155 | ME | 50 | 2 | 4 | Decreased libido on HRT | None | Testosterone added to HRT | Improvement | 6 |
| **Contraceptive Complications** | | | | | | | | | |
| 156 | BB | 31 | 0 | 0 | Amenorrhea on oral contraceptives | Pregnancy test: negative | Changed strength from 20 mg to 30 mg | Regular menses | 2 |
| 157 | VM | 63 | 5 | 5 | Postmenopausal bleeding IUD perforating through cervix | IUD culture: actinomycoses Endometrial biopsy: atrophic | IUD removal PCN G 500 qd × 4 wk | No recurrence | 6 |
| **Psychomatic Problems** | | | | | | | | | |
| None observed | | | | | | | | | |

**Example 12**

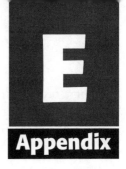

# E

**Appendix**

# Recommendations for Subspecialty Fellows

The pressing issue on most subspecialty fellows' minds is *when* to take their general boards exam. One thing for certain, you cannot sit for your subspecialty boards until you pass your general oral board exam. You will be horrified to acknowledge how much you have forgotten about your non-subspecialty areas. For this reason, I recommend you take your general board exam as soon as possible. The earliest is the second year of your fellowship. This means you need to start collecting cases on day one of the first year of your fellowship. I so hope you proactive folk are reading this now to remind you to save that doggone chief residency log for your non-specialty case list. It is a pathetic sight to witness a fellow discovering this after the fact. Finally, you can sit for your general board exam only once during your fellowship.

Since 2006, every page of your case list is stamped "fellow," so it's like there is a billboard with flashing lights announcing your title. Heck, it's pretty obvious, anyway, upon a mere glance of your case list by the type of cases. The most important tip to keep in mind is that you are sitting for the *general* boards, not your subspecialty boards. You are expected to have the same knowledge base in *all three* areas as any other candidate.

Undoubtedly your clinical acumen in your subspecialty will be above and beyond what is expected for the general boards. But the goal is not to verify your expertise in your subspecialty; your time will come when you sit for your subspecialty boards. The emphasis is on the areas unrelated to your subspecialty.

Therefore, starting now, spend no further time on studying your sub-specialty. Your energy should be diverted to refreshing your grasp of the basics in the other areas you used to know. Prioritize studying the topics that you know are going to be on the test. The list is as follows:

"Know cold" topics—Chapter 8, Table 1

"Hot" topics—Chapter 8, Table 2

Past "cases of the day"—Chapter 7, Tables 1, 2, and 3

Limiting your studying to these topics alone will cover at least 80% of your exam.

Traditionally, the base for patient management questions stems from the case list. Although you will certainly have some questions from the case list, it is not emphasized as much because the board has allowed fellows to submit a case list from their chief year in their non-subspecialty. It still must include 20 hospitalized or surgical patients as well as the office prac-tice case list. The cases must cover a spectrum of depth and variety within your subspecialty. Even though your case list may be limited, you will still be examined in all three areas: obstetrics, gynecology, and office practice.

While studying, keep in mind that you need to know only the basics to pass the question. You have become accustomed to knowing even the most trivial minutiae and groundbreaking research in your subspecialty. Refrain from trying to achieve the same depth in the general topics. Not only will you waste precious time, but you do not get extra credit for going beyond the required threshold.

The general exam is quite humbling. You are well respected and recog-nized for your expertise in your subspecialty. You know a lot about one area; now you need to know a little about everything again. It is amazing how much you have forgotten about the other areas.

There are only two reasons that a fellow fails the general board exam. The first is a pompous, "know-it-all" attitude. The fellow cannot resist belittling the examiner and debating with him at the same or higher level on the fellow's subspecialty topic. The second reason is failure to demon-strate the minimal knowledge base in non-subspecialty topics.

In conclusion, remember that you are taking your general boards. You need to demonstrate the same knowledge base in all three areas as any other candidate. No extra credit is given for going above and beyond the mandatory threshold, but certainly you will fail if you do not know your basics. Do not be arrogant and demeaning. Swallow your pride, and join the ranks with the generalists.

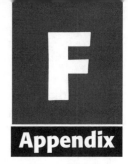

**Appendix**

# Recommendations for Military Personnel

The primary reason for seeking board certification is probably the same for civilian and military physicians. Some incentives, however, are unique to the military. If you are board-certified, you receive a monthly bonus stipend. Furthermore, board certification influences your assignment of duty position and station. You are more likely to be assigned to a sought-after teaching facility if you board-certified. Certainly, board certification makes you marketable if you decide to leave the military.

Historically, military personnel enjoy an excellent track record. Statistically as a group, you have a nearly 100% pass rate. Are you better trained? I doubt it, since most of you were trained in civilian residencies. The explanation probably lies in the unique differences and challenges of practicing OB/GYN in the military.

It usually becomes obvious when you are defending your case list that you lack the support of both OB/GYN and other colleagues because of the omnipresent physician shortage in the military. Ancillary resources are restricted because of geographical limitations and shortages. Your patient population is different. Deployments, missions, and nontraditional job duties often influence timing and urgency for evaluation, management, and follow-up. Thus, you must be more creative, broad-based, resourceful, and independent than your civilian colleagues. Examiners love it!

The examiner can tell instantly that you are in the military from the name of the hospital on your affidavit sheet. An age-old debate is whether you should make it obvious by wearing your uniform to the exam. One school of thought says that you should not stand out, yet feedback from those who wore their uniforms is emphatically favorable. You are so used to wearing your uniform anyway that it is a comforting familiarity. Most civilians and especially you feel stuffy and artificial in a business suit that is otherwise the necessary attire.

The uniform also lends a second-nature military bearing of extreme professionalism (e.g., saying "ma'am" and "sir") that is not routinely bestowed on examiners. They relish this tremendous display of respect and professionalism. They cannot help but extend the same courtesy to you. Not only do they admire your devotion to duty, they also respect the additional challenges and hardships that you incur simply because you are a military physician. You will be taken aback when ABOG dignitaries, as well as your examiners, will thank *you* for serving our country.

I believe that military bearing and courtesy also make the oral exam format more familiar. You seem to be able to bear the brunt of interrogation a little more easily than civilians. If you are not comfortable with your training experience alone, you can take a mock oral exam offered at the October meeting of the ACOG Armed Forces district.

In summary, I say: Don't hide it, flaunt it! Of course, I need to disclose that I am a retired Army colonel, but my career was with the National Guard and Reserves. I do know **both** the civilian and military perspective. Having disclosed that, go with the winning tide and proudly acknowledge that you are in the military. Recall the impact of the first impression. No doubt, a uniformed physician will make the ultimate first expression. After all, the adage, "You never get a second chance to make a great first impression," is posted in the entry to the AMEDD school hall at Ft. Sam Houston, Texas!

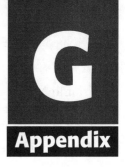

# Case List Review

We have discussed throughout the book the importance of having your case list reviewed. Of course, it is the most helpful **before** you turn it in on August 1. Your reviewers will pick up on not just the obvious but, equally important, the subtleties that can really add up. Ideally, you should have you case list reviewed in May and then in earlyJuly, after your first re-write.

The more reviews, the better. I recommend that your referring MFM review the Obstetrics case list; your GYN oncologist, your Gynecology case list; and your reproductive endocrinologist, your Office Practice case lists. The specialists represent those of your examiners and are especially important to help you recapture the specialist, rather than the generalist perspective.

Given, however, that this is your *general* boards, I recommend you have some generalists look at any of the three sections. Furthermore, you want to choose a stranger who is unfamiliar with your mode of practice, in order to give you a true unbiased picture. Finally, a non-medical person can pick up on typos and spelling errors.

Absolutely **all** of your reviewers should be clinicians. The practice of medicine is so dynamic that even one who only recently stopped practicing will already be out of date. This exam most definitely will hold you to the latest standards. Furthermore, your reviewer must also be performing the same surgeries and procedures as you in order to provide the most contemporary and comprehensive suggestions. You can sure bet your examiner is the expert for those as well.

Prior to August 1, the reviews are targeted to helping you strategically organize the case list to put your best foot forward. After August 1, the case list is cast in stone, and subsequent reviews help you defend your case list.

If you would like me to review your case list, please contact me.

A. Krishna Das, MD, FACOG
622 Sabine Drive
Hendersonville, NC 28739
(828) 692-2258
krisdas@earthlink.net
krisdas@mchsi.com

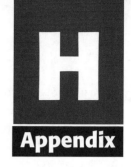

# America's OB/GYN
# Board Review Course

I discussed review courses in Chapter 4. I tried to present an objective list of criteria to aid in your selection of a course. I must disclose that I indeed have a bias for a particular course.

I have had the honor to lecture for a number of review courses over the past twenty years. I also have attended my fair share as well. This has afforded me the opportunity to become quite opinionated as to what I feel is the ideal course.

In 2007 I founded America's OB/GYN Board Review Course (ABC). I would like to go through that list from Chapter 4 and share why I designed ABC to be the ideal course. Admittedly, it is a constant work in progress, as we continue to raise the bar higher.

Our mission is to provide a review with *passion* and *compassion*. These are not words that I use lightly. At ABC, we want you to feel the energy and excitement about our absolute top notch personnel: the faculty, course director, and staff. There will be no question that excellence is the standard.

At the same time, there is a genuine sense of caring. You will not feel like just another number. The ABC staff want to understand *your* needs so we can best assist you. Customer service is second to none. We make a concerted effort to address each registrant by name. Your syllabus binder is customized with your name. The faculty is accessible and approachable, both during and *after* the course.

The course is five days. The duration was carefully researched based on registrant feedback. Five days is ideal to capture attention span and stamina.

You're just not used to sitting for hours on end listening to lectures anymore. Additionally, if you're barraged with so much material, you are overwhelmed with which topics to study first. The course is strategically held Wednesday to Sunday to minimize the time away from your practice and family. The course is offered both in the spring and the fall to best meet your strategic study needs.

The course syllabus is very strategically selected based *entirely* on what's on your test. Note our name is a **board** review course, not just a review course. ABC covers *90%* of the test topics in just five days. I carefully adjust the syllabus based on exam trends. As the course director, I choose and assign the topics to my faculty. This prevents the lectures from being laden with their research interest.

We claim to have only **wow** faculty. They are hand picked by me not only for their expertise, but especially for their finesse and charisma in public speaking. Typically the speaker's are subspecialists who will lecture on that topic *all day*. This allows them to cover more material quickly, as they never have to worry about duplicating what the speaker before covered. This also provides for a wonderful, nurturing student-teacher atmosphere. All the speakers must be clinicians. The test is a very clinical one, so your mentors must be alongside you in the trenches to truly empathize and understand the issues. They truly practice what they preach. You will find their pearls of wisdom helpful not only on the test but in your day-to-day practice as well.

The format of the lectures is strict. This is a clinical review in accordance with the ACOG standards. All speakers must blatantly point out, both verbally and in their handouts, the exam focus. Each registrant receives a manual listing each topic and the exam focus. This manual is designed to accompany and follow along as the topic is presented. It is printed on yellow pages, and we've repeatedly been told it is worth its weight in gold, as you can condense the 900-page binder onto this 55-page gem. Talk about bottom line up front!

Although the speakers are board certified, they must have a comprehensive and up-to-date understanding of the exam process. This book is mandatory reading, so they have a keen understanding of the whole oral exam process from start to finish. Additionally, the speakers are updated after each exam. All of the speakers regularly give mock oral exams themselves. At the end of the day, it should be crystal clear what is on your test. The lectures should provide sufficient detail such that you do not need to go beyond the syllabus for any more review of that topic.

Whereas the days are filled with didactic lectures, the evenings are filled with optional evening sessions on strategy and tactics. The spring courses focus on how to construct your case list. The fall courses focus on how to defend your case list. The faculty are available to provide mock oral exams, case list reviews, and our signature round robins of the structured cases.

I know most of you have never seen another case list beyond your own. Why reinvent the wheel when you can check out our case list library? We have scores of binders containing previous candidates' case lists. They are filled with a wide array of teaching points. You can follow a case list from its genesis, with recordings of the review and with recommendations and tip both on constructing and defending your case list. You can then view the updated drafts incorporating these changes all the way to the final product. Some of the case lists even have the actual questions that were asked during the exam. A few minutes browsing through the case list library will save you oodles of precious time later.

Understandably, you may be a bit saturated by the evening. Thus, ABC also offers full-day workshops on case list construction as well as oral exam strategy. They are available the day before the courses or throughout the year in locations throughout the country.

We are sensitive to the financial constraints of residents and new practitioners. We offer discounts for residents/fellows, signing up with a friend, returning registrants, and the military. We aggressively negotiate with the hotels to provide a luxurious environment conducive to learning, but at a modest price. We demand that they honor our compassion and passion theme as well. You will find above-and-beyond features such as suites, shuttles to nearby restaurants, grocery stores, drug stores, etc. All our hotels must have a fitness center to nurture your physical needs so your mind can work better. We even negotiate complimentary Internet access so you can stay in touch with your home or office. Finally, there are no hidden expenses. The hotel provides a complimentary shuttle from the airport. Breakfast, lunch, and snacks are included in your registration fee. The ultimate financial aid is our money-back guarantee in the unlikely event that you do not pass your boards. I am not aware that *any other* course has the same offer or seal of confidence.

By the way, for you proactive folks who are still preparing for your written board exam, ABC can help you too. We have workshops geared specifically for the written test, with tips on how to increase your score. For those who have failed, we provide the only course that has education specialists who can analyze your performance and recommend corrective steps.

Additionally, ABC has computerized tests with questions modeled after the written board format to simulate your exam.

I strongly encourage you to attend. There is something to be said for stepping away from it all in order to channel your undivided attention to your studies for five days. However, the course is available on DVDs and CDs should you be unable to attend or if you simply want to reinforce the lectures.

I encourage you to compare ABC to other review courses. I think we have created the ideal course. We take pride in preparing you for *every step* of your board examination quest: your written, oral, and recertification exams. I invite you to check us out at **www.americasboardreview.com**. Please feel free to call us at 1-877-ABC-OBGYN (1-877-222-6249). I invite your suggestions and comments. As always, you are welcome to contact me at krisdas@earthlink.net or krisdas@mchsi.com.

# Index

**247**